Advanced Technologies in Vascular Neurosurgery

Erol Veznedaroglu
Editor

Advanced Technologies in Vascular Neurosurgery

Techniques, Controversies and New Paradigms

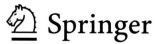 Springer

Editor
Erol Veznedaroglu
Department of Neurosurgery
Drexel University School of Medicine
Philadelphia, PA, USA

Global Neurosciences Institute
Pennington, NJ, USA

ISBN 978-3-031-67491-4   ISBN 978-3-031-67492-1   (eBook)
https://doi.org/10.1007/978-3-031-67492-1

This Springer imprint is published by the registered company Springer Nature Switzerland AG
The registered company address is: Gewerbestrasse 11, 6330 Cham, Switzerland

If disposing of this product, please recycle the paper.

This text is dedicated first and always to my family, the sacrifice of our work rests solely on our families. My wife, Elisabeth, who has supported the crazy life of a Vascular Neurosurgeon for 30 years, and my amazing vchildren, Lauren and Alec, who have been an inspiration and joy.

This year we lost a true Pioneer and Legend—Dr L Nick Hopkins MD.
Dr Hopkins saw what none of us did 40 years ago. As all visionaries do, he suffered by challenging the status quo and fighting to show a better way to treat our patients.
Dr Hopkins was the first to open the door of endovascular

therapy as "Brain Surgery" and learn from our partners in Cardiology and Interventional Radiology. This book, and indeed our specialty, would not be possible if it were not for him. Nick was a mentor, friend, and inspiration to all those who were lucky enough to know him. The three "Nick Wisdoms" I remember as a medical student and live by:

Why Not?, If you're not making waves you're not doing anything worthwhile, Expletive em

Preface

For the first time in the history of medicine, technology has outpaced our ability to use it. There is very little that cannot be achieved due to lack of technology; the paradigm shift now is what should we be doing with it. The brain remains the last frontier in medicine where we still lack full understanding of its function and vast neural network. This allows for the perfect marriage of technology and discovery for better outcomes and cures of disorders of the nervous system. The ability to access virtually every area of the brain via the cerebrovasculature has never been more important.

This flood of new technology, including artificial intelligence, brings with it challenges of how best to use it in modern practice. Vascular Neurosurgery has undergone seismic shifts in the last decade. The ability to access the cerebrovascular through a small puncture in the groin or wrist has opened up safe, less-invasive, and better outcomes for previously untreatable conditions. Indeed, endovascular treatment has now become a new option for brain tumors, subdural hematomas, and even intracranial hypertension. The old adage "just because you can do something doesn't mean you should" has never been more true. The tried and true also has a critical role in this new dawn; however, maintaining basic skills will be more of an issue.

The goal of this text is to expose the new technological advances in a comprehensive and balanced way. As we have learned countless times in modern medicine, new is not always better and in fact may be dangerous. The ability to asses newer techniques in a way that is always in the patients' best interest is the ultimate goal. In this text, leaders in the field of Vascular Neurosurgery will discuss this new technology as well as the controversies it raises. The reader will have an unbiased and comprehensive exposure to the latest innovations and how they are currently being used.

Philadelphia, PA USA   Erol Veznedaroglu

Contents

1 The Future of Neurointervention: New Procedures, New Practitioners, and New Problems 1
Andre Monteiro, William Metcalf-Doetsch,
Wasiq I. Khawar, Adnan H. Siddiqui, and Elad I. Levy

2 Minimally Invasive Intracerebral Hemorrhage Removal 27
Jack Jestus, Demi Dawkins, Kenneth Moore,
Adam Arthur, and Christopher Nickele

3 Middle Meningeal Artery Embolization for Chronic Subdural Hematoma 51
Alina Mohanty and Peter Kan

4 Role of Bypass in the Modern Era: Technological Advancements in Adjuncts for EC-IC Bypass 61
Sanjana Salwi, Visish Srinivasan,
and Jan-Karl Burkhardt

5 Embolic Protection Devices for Carotid Artery Stenting: Where Is the Evidence? 71
Mohanad Sulaiman and Mandy J. Binning

6 Closing the Gap: Addressing the Lag in Stroke Care Evolution 87
Erol Veznedaroglu, Karen Greenberg,
and Haley Fitzgerald

7   Venous Sinus Stenting for Idiopathic
Intracranial Hypertension 103
Justin M. Cappuzzo, Steven B. Housley,
Muhammad Waqas, Andre Monteiro,
Ryan M. Hess, Elad I. Levy, and Adnan H. Siddiqui

8   Robotic-Assisted Endovascular Intervention 135
Marcus Wong and Gavin Britz

9   Present Rationale and Future Directions
for Intracranial Aneurysm Screening
and Rupture Risk Prediction: The Road
to Precision Surgery for Intracranial Aneurysms ... 147
Abhijith R. Bathini, Maged Ghoche,
Seyed Farzad Maroufi, Brandon A. Nguyen,
Maria José Pachón-Londoño, Ataollah Shahbandi,
Devi P. Patra, and Bernard R. Bendok

10 Endovascular Management and Treatment
of Acute Ischemic Stroke 177
Omer Doron, Yafell Serulle, Likowsky L. Desir,
Hamza Khilji, and Rafael Ortiz

Index 239

Contributors

Adam Arthur Neurosurgery, University of Tennessee Health Science Center, Memphis, TN, USA

Neurosurgery, Semmes Murphey Clinic, Memphis, TN, United States

Abhijith R. Bathini Department of Neurological Surgery, Mayo Clinic, Phoenix, AZ, USA

Neurosurgery Simulation and Innovation Lab, Mayo Clinic, Phoenix, AZ, USA

Bernard R. Bendok Department of Neurological Surgery, Mayo Clinic, Phoenix, AZ, USA

Neurosurgery Simulation and Innovation Lab, Mayo Clinic, Phoenix, AZ, USA

Mayo Clinic Alix School of Medicine, Scottsdale, AZ, USA

Precision Neuro-therapeutics Innovation Lab, Mayo Clinic, Phoenix, AZ, USA

Department of Otolaryngology-Head & Neck Surgery, Mayo Clinic, Phoenix, AZ, USA

Department of Radiology, Mayo Clinic, Phoenix, AZ, USA

Mandy J. Binning Global Neurosciences Institute (GNI), Drexel University, Pennington, NJ, USA

Gavin Britz Department of Neurosurgery, Houston Methodist Neurological Institute, Houston, TX, USA

Jan-Karl Burkhardt University of Pennsylvania, Department of Neurosurgery, Philadelphia, PA, USA

Justin M. Cappuzzo Department of Neurosurgery, Jacobs School of Medicine and Biomedical Sciences, University at Buffalo, Buffalo, NY, USA

Department of Neurosurgery, Gates Vascular Institute at Kaleida Health, Buffalo, NY, USA

Demi Dawkins Neurosurgery, Semmes Murphey Clinic, Memphis, TN, United States

Likowsky L. Desir Department of Neurosurgery, Lenox Hill Hospital, Donald and Barbara Zucker School of Medicine at Hofstra/Northwell Health, New York, NY, USA

Omer Doron Department of Neurosurgery, Lenox Hill Hospital, Donald and Barbara Zucker School of Medicine at Hofstra/Northwell Health, New York, NY, USA

Haley Fitzgerald Department of Neurosurgery, Global Neurosciences Institute, Pennington, NJ, USA

Maged Ghoche Department of Neurological Surgery, Mayo Clinic, Phoenix, AZ, USA

Neurosurgery Simulation and Innovation Lab, Mayo Clinic, Phoenix, AZ, USA

Karen Greenberg Departments of Clinical Education, Emergency Medicine, Neurosurgery, Drexel University School of Medicine, Philadelphia, PA, USA

Department of Neurology, Temple Lewis Katz School of Medicine, Philadelphia, PA, USA

Ryan M. Hess Department of Neurosurgery, Jacobs School of Medicine and Biomedical Sciences, University at Buffalo, Buffalo, NY, USA

Department of Neurosurgery, Gates Vascular Institute at Kaleida Health, Buffalo, NY, USA

Steven B. Housley Department of Neurosurgery, Jacobs School of Medicine and Biomedical Sciences, University at Buffalo, Buffalo, NY, USA

Department of Neurosurgery, Gates Vascular Institute at Kaleida Health, Buffalo, NY, USA

Jack Jestus Neurosurgery, University of Tennessee Health Science Center, Memphis, TN, USA

Peter Kan Neurosurgery, The University of Texas Medical Branch at Galveston, Galveston, TX, USA

Wasiq I. Khawar Department of Neurosurgery, Jacobs School of Medicine and Biomedical Sciences, University at Buffalo, Buffalo, NY, USA

Hamza Khilji Department of Neurosurgery, Lenox Hill Hospital, Donald and Barbara Zucker School of Medicine at Hofstra/ Northwell Health, New York, NY, USA

Elad I. Levy Department of Neurosurgery, Jacobs School of Medicine and Biomedical Sciences, University at Buffalo, Buffalo, NY, USA

Department of Neurosurgery, Gates Vascular Institute at Kaleida Health, Buffalo, NY, USA

Department of Radiology, Jacobs School of Medicine and Biomedical Sciences, University at Buffalo, Buffalo, NY, USA

Canon Stroke and Vascular Research Center, University at Buffalo, Buffalo, NY, USA

Jacobs Institute, Buffalo, NY, USA

Seyed Farzad Maroufi Tehran University of Medical Sciences, Tehran, Iran

William Metcalf-Doetsch Department of Neurosurgery, Jacobs School of Medicine and Biomedical Sciences, University at Buffalo, Buffalo, NY, USA

Department of Neurosurgery, Gates Vascular Institute at Kaleida Health, Buffalo, NY, USA

Alina Mohanty Baylor College of Medicine Department of Neurosurgery, Houston, TX, USA

Andre Monteiro Department of Neurosurgery, Jacobs School of Medicine and Biomedical Sciences, University at Buffalo, Buffalo, NY, USA

Department of Neurosurgery, Gates Vascular Institute at Kaleida Health, Buffalo, NY, USA

Kenneth Moore Neurosurgery, University of Tennessee Health Science Center, Memphis, TN, USA

Neurosurgery, Semmes Murphey Clinic, Memphis, TN, United States

Brandon A. Nguyen Department of Neurological Surgery, Mayo Clinic, Phoenix, AZ, USA

Neurosurgery Simulation and Innovation Lab, Mayo Clinic, Phoenix, AZ, USA

Mayo Clinic Alix School of Medicine, Scottsdale, AZ, USA

Christopher Nickele Neurosurgery, University of Tennessee Health Science Center, Memphis, TN, USA

Neurosurgery, Semmes Murphey Clinic, Memphis, TN, United States

Rafael Ortiz Department of Neurosurgery, Lenox Hill Hospital, Donald and Barbara Zucker School of Medicine at Hofstra/Northwell Health, New York, NY, USA

Maria José Pachón-Londoño Department of Neurological Surgery, Mayo Clinic, Phoenix, AZ, USA

Neurosurgery Simulation and Innovation Lab, Mayo Clinic, Phoenix, AZ, USA

Devi P. Patra Department of Neurological Surgery, Mayo Clinic, Phoenix, AZ, USA

Neurosurgery Simulation and Innovation Lab, Mayo Clinic, Phoenix, AZ, USA

Sanjana Salwi University of Pennsylvania, Department of Neurosurgery, Philadelphia, PA, USA

Yafell Serulle Department of Neurosurgery, Lenox Hill Hospital, Donald and Barbara Zucker School of Medicine at Hofstra/Northwell Health, New York, NY, USA

Ataollah Shahbandi Tehran University of Medical Sciences, Tehran, Iran

Adnan H. Siddiqui Department of Neurosurgery, Jacobs School of Medicine and Biomedical Sciences, University at Buffalo, Buffalo, NY, USA

Department of Neurosurgery, Gates Vascular Institute at Kaleida Health, Buffalo, NY, USA

Department of Radiology, Jacobs School of Medicine and Biomedical Sciences, University at Buffalo, Buffalo, NY, USA

Canon Stroke and Vascular Research Center, University at Buffalo, Buffalo, NY, USA

Jacobs Institute, Buffalo, NY, USA

Visish Srinivasan University of Pennsylvania, Department of Neurosurgery, Philadelphia, PA, USA

Mohanad Sulaiman Global Neurosciences Institute (GNI), Drexel University, Pennington, NJ, USA

Erol Veznedaroglu Department of Neurosurgery, Drexel University School of Medicine, Philadelphia, PA, USA

Global Neurosciences Institute, Pennington, NJ, USA

Muhammad Waqas Department of Neurosurgery, Jacobs School of Medicine and Biomedical Sciences, University at Buffalo, Buffalo, NY, USA

Department of Neurosurgery, Gates Vascular Institute at Kaleida Health, Buffalo, NY, USA

Marcus Wong Department of Neurosurgery, Houston Methodist Neurological Institute, Houston, TX, USA

The Future of Neurointervention: New Procedures, New Practitioners, and New Problems

Andre Monteiro, William Metcalf-Doetsch, Wasiq I. Khawar, Adnan H. Siddiqui, and Elad I. Levy

Abbreviations and Acronyms (Please note that the study acronyms have not been expanded in the text)

ADL	Activities of daily living
AIS	Acute ischemic stroke(s)
BCI	Brain-computer interface(s)
BGC	Balloon guide catheter
CSF	Cerebrospinal fluid
CSFVF	Cerebrospinal fluid-venous fistula

A. Monteiro · W. Metcalf-Doetsch
Department of Neurosurgery, Jacobs School of Medicine and Biomedical Sciences, University at Buffalo, Buffalo, NY, USA

Department of Neurosurgery, Gates Vascular Institute at Kaleida Health, Buffalo, NY, USA
e-mail: amonteiro@ubns.com

W. I. Khawar
Department of Neurosurgery, Jacobs School of Medicine and Biomedical Sciences, University at Buffalo, Buffalo, NY, USA

DAWN   DWI or CTP Assessment with Clinical
                    Mismatch in the Triage of Wake-Up and
                    Late Presenting Strokes Undergoing
                    Neurointervention with Trevo
DEFUSE 3   Endovascular Therapy Following Imaging
                    Evaluation for Ischemic Stroke 3
DEVT   Direct Endovascular Thrombectomy vs.
                    Combined IVT and Endovascular
                    Thrombectomy for Patients with Acute
                    Large Vessel Occlusion in the Anterior
                    Circulation
DIRECT-MT   Direct Intra-arterial thrombectomy in
                    order to Revascularize AIS patients with
                    large vessel occlusions Efficiently in
                    Chinese Tertiary Hospitals: a Multicenter
                    randomized clinical Trial
ESCAPE   Endovascular treatment for Small Core
                    and Anterior circulation Proximal occlu-
                    sion with Emphasis on minimizing CT to
                    recanalization times
ETCHES I   Endovascular Treatment of
                    Communicating Hydrocephalus with the
                    eShunt System
EXTEND IA   Extending the Time for Thrombolysis
                    in Emergency Neurological Deficits—
                    Intra-arterial

A. H. Siddiqui · E. I. Levy (✉)
Department of Neurosurgery, Jacobs School of Medicine and
Biomedical Sciences, University at Buffalo, Buffalo, NY, USA

Department of Neurosurgery, Gates Vascular Institute at Kaleida Health,
Buffalo, NY, USA

Department of Radiology, Jacobs School of Medicine and Biomedical
Sciences, University at Buffalo, Buffalo, NY, USA

Canon Stroke and Vascular Research Center, University at Buffalo,
Buffalo, NY, USA

Jacobs Institute, Buffalo, NY, USA
e-mail: asiddiqui@ubns.com; editorial@ubns.com; elevy@ubns.com

F	French
h	Hour
IIH	Idiopathic intracranial hypertension
LVO	Large vessel occlusion
MR CLEAN	Multicenter Randomized Clinical Trial of Endovascular Treatment for Acute Ischemic Stroke in the Netherlands
MR CLEAN-NO IV	Multicenter Randomized Clinical trial of Endovascular treatment for Acute ischemic stroke in the Netherlands investigating the added benefit of intravenous alteplase prior to intra-arterial thrombectomy in stroke patients with an intracranial occlusion of the anterior circulation
MRI	Magnetic resonance imaging
MT	Mechanical thrombectomy
NINDS	National Institute of Neurological Disorders and Stroke
REVASCAT	Randomized Trial of Revascularization with Solitaire FR Device versus Best Medical Therapy in the Treatment of Acute Stroke Due to Anterior Occlusion Circulation Large Vessel Occlusion Presenting within Eight Hours of Symptomatic Onset
SAH	Subarachnoid hemorrhage
SKIP	Direct Mechanical Thrombectomy in Acute LVO Stroke
SWIFT PRIME	Solitaire With the Intention For Thrombectomy as PRIMary Endovascular treatment
TFA	Transfemoral approach(es)
tPA	Tissue plasminogen activator
TRA	Transfemoral approach(es)
US	United States
VSS	Venous sinus stenting

Introduction

Neurointervention is a thriving and dynamic specialty whose practitioners are actively forging new paths and championing revolutionary new therapies. Many of these procedures are providing minimally invasive treatment alternatives in lieu of historic open surgical options or adjunctive surgical therapies. In reflection of the exponential growth potential, the number of trainees in neurointervention is also increasing to provide sufficient coverage and availability of these novel therapies to patients. Several challenges arise hand in hand with a constantly shifting landscape of innovative therapies and new devices for endovascular practitioners who must also be skilled in the systems- and practice-based implementation of these advancements in patient populations. This chapter describes the benefits and obstacles originating from this fast-paced environment, examines some of the newest procedures and training requirements, and discusses challenges facing the neuroendovascular field in pushing the frontier of cerebrovascular disease treatment.

New Problems

Fast-Paced Evolution of Technology

Perhaps the greatest challenge for neurointerventionists of both younger and older generations is also the most exciting aspect of this field: the fast-paced evolution of technologies, treatments available, and indications.

Acute Ischemic Stroke Paradigm Shift

No other area in the realm of cerebrovascular intervention has so clearly a stand-out history of innovation in new procedures and devices as stroke and ischemic disease. Until nearly 8 years ago, intravenous alteplase was the first-line modality for most acute ischemic strokes (AIS), a therapeutic strategy that had been unchanged since the NINDS trials in 1995 [1]. Although many endovascular modalities for recanalization were available since then, it took two decades to firmly establish the superiority of these techniques over medical therapy [1, 2]. As a joint effort within the global neurointervention community, the publication of multiple randomized trials in 2015 (MR CLEAN, ESCAPE, REVASCAT, SWIFT PRIME, and EXTEND IA) dramatically changed the treatment scenario for AIS [3]. Mechanical thrombectomy (MT) with stent retrievers became the gold standard treatment for AIS due to anterior large vessel occlusion (LVO) for patients presenting within early time windows. With the assistance of perfusion imaging, the MT window also rapidly changed toward the present 24-hour therapeutic window for selected patients based on the results of the DAWN and DEFUSE 3 trials published in 2018 [4–6]. Furthermore, the development of more flexible and navigable large-bore distal aspiration catheters introduced equipoise between the use of these devices and the established stent retrievers, with subsequent randomized trials reporting noninferiority of one device over another [7]. Stent retrievers and distal aspiration catheters have undergone technological evolution to miniaturized and adjustable-expansion versions to keep up with ongoing debates about endovascular treatment of smaller vessels (i.e., distal and medium vessel occlusions). Present debates also exist regarding the use of newer generation balloon guide catheters (BGCs) to arrest flow and minimize clot fragmentation and distal embolization, which have been largely adopted due to their better flexibility, versatility, and navigability in comparison to older generation BGCs [8–13]. Although these few examples represent the astounding technological advancement that requires trainees and operators to be up to date with their skills and options, there are even more radical paradigm shifts in discussion. The benefit of intravenous thrombolysis, as aforementioned to have once been the first-line treatment for all AIS, is now in question for LVO patients after the publication of the results of four randomized trials (SKIP, DEVT, DIRECT-MT, and MR CLEAN-NO IV) comparing MT alone versus MT plus intravenous alteplase [14–17]. All these robust changes not only create challenges to trainees, established operators, and researchers but also signal the evolution of the field as a whole toward improving patient care through evidence-based practice.

Variety of Endovascular Therapies for Intracranial Aneurysms

Endovascular management of intracranial aneurysms has made considerable progress since coils were the only available technology [18]. The times of microsurgical clipping versus coiling are essentially gone as technology evolved and the field matured with the acceptance of endovascular neurosurgery within its practice. Intracranial laser-cut stents were developed to provide the ability to safely treat wide-necked aneurysms without the risk of coil prolapse [19]. Although the earlier generation of these devices had limitations, such as kinking or fracture in sharp curvatures, the most recent laser-cut and braided microstents have mostly overcome these issues [20]. Perhaps the most remarkable evolution of endovascular neurosurgery within the last decades was the advent of flow diverters. These devices have shifted the landscape of internal carotid artery aneurysm treatment toward endovascular management [21]. Aneurysms of the posterior circulation have presented more challenges, but flow diversion is slowly becoming the mainstay of treatment at this location as well [22]. Furthermore, industries are exploring surface-modification and bioabsorbable technologies to reduce the need for antiplatelet therapy and diminish the thrombogenic potential of these devices, which may improve the quality of life of patients with unruptured aneurysms treated with these devices and even unlock many possibilities in the treatment of ruptured aneurysms with complex morphologies [23, 24]. The most recent class of intracranial devices are the intrasaccular flow disruptors, such as the Woven EndoBridge device (Terumo), which can potentially eliminate the need for antiplatelet therapy and have promising applications in the setting of subarachnoid hemorrhage (SAH) [25]. Similarly, temporary expandable neck-bridging stents, such as the Comaneci (Rapid Medical), have provided the option of assisting coil packing of ruptured aneurysms without the need to permanently deploy a stent in the parent vessel (thereby eliminating the need for antiplatelet therapy) or occlude the parent vessel lumen (such as during balloon-assisted coiling) [26].

Presently, excellence in cerebrovascular care can only be achieved through a patient-first approach, with an understanding that microsurgery and all the new endovascular modalities complement each other and should be applied in appropriate situations [27]. Such a change in the field also creates certain "pressure" that aspiring or younger cerebrovascular surgeons should pursue hybrid training to provide comprehensive options to their patients. Therefore, all the innovation encourages younger and older operators alike to be familiar with novel technical nuances and seek appropriate applications for each technology, keeping a balance between the zeal exuded by industry and the actual benefit to patients.

New Practitioners

Awareness of Demand and Treatment Disparities for Acute Ischemic Stroke

Along with the expansion of treatment possibilities through neurointervention combined with the high incidence and prevalence of cerebrovascular diseases, a growing demand for new practitioners was anticipated. Presently, AIS care is perhaps the most affected area of neurointervention regarding demand and growth of centers. Therefore, in this section, we focus on relevant discussions about present and future directions of AIS care.

Stroke care is changing not only within the "micro" aspect of individual patient treatments but also in the "macro" organizational and certification aspects of clinical practice. Given the paradigm shift toward endovascular-based management of AIS, improvements must target better and wider direct access to MT-capable centers. Transportation of patient directly to MT-capable centers, bypassing those without endovascular capability, can increase the coverage of timely access to MT by approximately 10% [28]. However, a recent study by Aldstadt et al. that was based on data from 1944 stroke centers obtained from the list of Joint Commission-accredited facilities reported a great lack of

coverage and disparity in timely MT access within the USA
(Fig. 1.1) [29]. Access to MT-capable centers within 1 hour (h)
was the case for approximately 50% of the population by ground
transportation and 65% if ground and air transportation were
combined. This corresponded to 113 million residents without 1-h
access to an MT-capable center by air or ground. Furthermore,
such lack of timely access was not evenly distributed across the
USA, with coverage ranging from 0% to more than 80% of inhab-
itants, depending on the state where the event occurred.

With such a great demand for more neurointerventionists,
maintaining the quality of treatment delivered is of paramount
importance. The threshold for the volume of cases to obtain
accreditation in thrombectomy centers is under debate [30–33].
Many defend that thresholds should be raised to ensure
competency in patient care, as recent studies have demonstrated

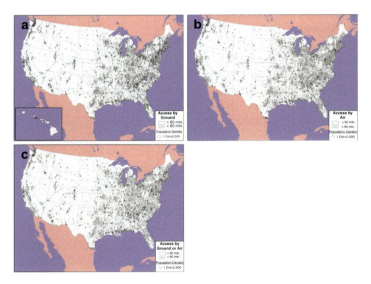

Fig. 1.1 US maps showing 60-minute access to endovascular-capable stroke
care centers (ECCs) with respect to population density. Each dot represents a
2500-resident census block. The gray area indicates 60-minute coverage via
ground (**a**), air (**b**), and ground or air (**c**). (With permission from Aldstadt
et al. [29])

that case volume matters more than accreditation status [30–33]. Therefore, the bright future of stroke care is attributable not only to technological advancements but also to the dedication of operators to maintain the quality of training during an overwhelming evolution in a short period of time while also providing these benefits to the largest number of patients possible.

New Impactful Skill Sets

As mentioned earlier, the fast evolution of the neurointervention field creates additional challenges related to new skill sets to be learned and mastered. In this section, we briefly discuss novel skill sets that may have an impact on the practice of neurointervention, especially for new practitioners.

The Transradial Wave

Neurointervention is considered by many to be in its "childhood" when compared to the "older" field of interventional cardiology. Among the many lessons and tools that were brought from that field, radial artery access was adapted more than 20 years ago as an alternative to transfemoral approach (TFA) in selected patients [34]. However, it was only recently that transradial approaches (TRA) gained popularity among neurointerventionists [35–38]. Arguments favoring a shift toward a "radial-first"-based practice are the lower rate of access site complications (e.g., less hematomas), less painful recovery, and earlier ambulation [36–38]. Several case series reported in the literature provide evidence of the feasibility, safety, and effectiveness of TRA for aneurysm treatments (e.g., coiling and variations, flow diversion, and intrasaccular flow disruption; embolizations for subdural hematomas, arteriovenous malformations, and fistulas; and stenting procedures for extracranial and intracranial atherosclerotic stenosis) [39]. Such a paradigm shift has even motivated industry to develop better and optimized catheters specifically for anatomy pertinent to the TRA route [36]. This change in practice created a whole new horizon of technical skill set to be learned and optimized by trainees and operators [37]. Although TRA have been shown to be as safe, feasible, and effective as TFA for most procedures, it is important to note that controversies still remain regarding this approach in the treatment of stroke [9].

Concomitantly with the rise of TRA, the use of BGCs for MT was also highlighted in the literature [11]. Flow arrest provided by BGCs during MT was shown to increase the rate of first-pass recanalization and potentially reduce the rate of clot fragmentation and distal migration, therefore also improving the rate of complete recanalization [8, 13]. However, given the smaller size of the radial artery, MT through TRA was being performed mostly with 6- or 7-French (F) catheters, not allowing the use of BGCs, which have 8-F diameters [9, 12]. Therefore, concerns were raised about the use of TRA for MT in a study by Siddiqui et al. that demonstrated lower rates of successful reperfusion and worst clinical outcomes with TRA in comparison to TFA for MT [9]. More recently, the same group reported an alternative solution, describing a technique that uses sheathless insertion of an 8-F BGC through the radial artery during MT [10, 12]. The technique was successful mostly in cases with radial artery diameters larger than 2.5 mm, and there were no access site complications. This technique has not been compared directly to TFA with BGC. In summary, TRA is an essential part of the skill set of modern neurointerventionists, with potential to add to their practice if wisely used.

Robotics

The first robotic neuroendovascular intervention performed in a human patient was reported in 2020 [40]. Although such technology is in its infancy, such advancement may have implications for the practice of neurointervention in the near future [41]. Robot-assisted endovascular procedures are approved for percutaneous coronary and peripheral vascular interventions but not widely used yet [41]. A few limitations still exist, such as the complexity of cases that can be performed and the elevated cost associated with the technology in the absence of appropriate cost-effective studies. Given that present robotic systems do not provide tactile feedback, treatment of delicate anatomy is not optimal or entirely

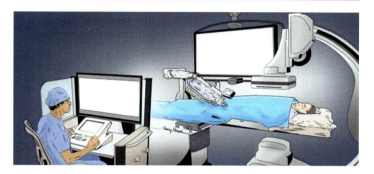

Fig. 1.2 Illustration of a robotic neurointervention setup in which the operator is not exposed to radiation

safe given that operators rely on this feedback to perform complex procedures [41]. Furthermore, one of the main arguments supporting the use of robotics is to reduce radiation exposure to operators (Fig. 1.2) [40, 41]. However, an interventional team is required in the operating room for completion of robotic procedures; therefore, the radiation hazard is not entirely eliminated [41]. Nevertheless, trainee education in robotic neurointervention is already a reality at a few centers. Furthermore, this will become an important skill set to be acquired if implementation of robotics is successful in promoting remote access to MT and other procedures in distant and underserved areas.

New Procedures

Certain diseases never thought to be manageable with neurointervention have become targets for this treatment modality after mechanisms of these conditions have been further elucidated or multidisciplinary collaborations have merged endovascular technology with new possibilities. In this section, we briefly discuss a few selected new procedures that challenge previous assumptions of management.

Cerebrospinal Fluid-Venous Fistula Embolization for Intracranial Hypotension

With advancements in digital subtraction myelography and decubitus computed tomography myelography, cerebrospinal fluid-venous fistulas (CSFVFs) became more detectable and have been increasingly recognized as a more prevalent cause of intracranial hypotension than previously thought [42]. These fistulas are abnormal connections between the CSF within the subarachnoid space and the venous drainage system, more often occurring at spinal levels [43, 44]. It is thought that these connections may occur due to rupture of arachnoid granulations into the paraspinal veins through diverticula of the dura that form the nerve root sheaths, creating direct CSF flow into the venous circulation and, consequently, CSF depletion and intracranial hypotension (Fig. 1.3) [43, 44]. Previous modalities of treatment for CSFVF included fibrin glue or a blood patch, nerve root skeletonization, and surgical ligation. Surgical ligation is highly effective because it definitively disconnects the venous outflow from the thecal sac [45]. However, it is a surgical procedure with all the risks inherent to invasive treatments, such as surgical wound infections and injury to surrounding structures. Therefore, minimally invasive alternatives with better effectiveness than fibrin glue or a blood patch are desirable [44].

Recently, Brinjikji et al. described CSFVF embolization as a novel therapy for intracranial hypotension [43]. The paraspinal veins are reached via microcatheter navigation to the azygos vein coming from the superior vena cava, and Onyx (Medtronic) is then injected to form a cast within the paraspinal, intercostal, foraminal, lateral epidural, and intersegmental veins [46]. Onyx 18 was preferably used given its higher penetration, and a plug of Onyx 34 can be inserted to prevent reflux of the Onyx 18; however, Borg et al. reported the use of a balloon microcatheter for that purpose [44, 46]. The largest series reported by Brinjikji et al. comprised 40 patients in which 50 CSFVFs were embolized, with improvement of clinical symptoms and magnetic resonance imaging (MRI) findings (e.g., brain sagging, pachymeningeal enhancement) experienced by 90% of the patients [44]. The most common postprocedural

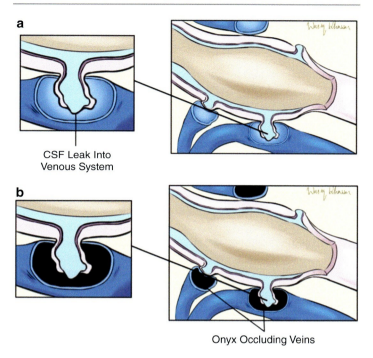

a

CSF Leak Into
Venous System

b

Onyx Occluding Veins

Fig. 1.3 Possible explanation for cerebrospinal fluid (CSF) fistulas, in which an arachnoid granulation into a dural diverticula in the nerve root sheath results in a CSF leak into the venous circulation (**a**). After embolization, the Onyx (Medtronic) cast occludes the leakage site (**b**)

finding was pain localized to the injection site, which tended to improve over a few weeks without the need of medication in 30% of the patients. Interestingly, "rebound" intracranial hypertension was seen in 17.5% of patients. This finding raised discussion by the authors regarding a possible relationship between intracranial hypotension and undiagnosed idiopathic intracranial hypotension [44]. Although CSFVF embolization appears to be the most effective and safe minimally invasive treatment for intracranial hypotension so far, future larger series will determine whether this therapy will become a mainstay of management.

Venous Sinus Stenting for Idiopathic Intracranial Hypertension

Idiopathic intracranial hypertension (IIH) affects 19 per 100,000 women who are between the age of 20 and 44 years and are at least 20% above their ideal body weight [47]. The etiology of this condition remains elusive, but it is presently accepted that impaired cerebrospinal fluid (CSF) dynamics is a main feature of the disease. Theories to explain this abnormality are that truncal obesity may result in central venous hypertension that builds up to the intracranial sinuses, reducing CSF absorption in the arachnoid granulations. Furthermore, studies in recent years have observed that venous sinus stenosis can be present in up to 93% of IIH patients [48]. This feature is hypothesized to be a consequence of increased intracranial pressure that causes collapse of the venous sinuses at vulnerable segments, such as the transverse-sigmoid junction [49–53]. A collapsed sinus would then worsen the intra-cranial hypertension in the segments distal to the stenotic seg-ment, further perpetuating a reduction in CSF absorption and an increase in intracranial pressure [54].

In patients with evidence of sinus stenosis in whom IIH is refractory to medical management and CSF diversion, venous sinus stenting (VSS) has arisen as a promising treatment [55]. The first case was reported in 2002 by Higgins et al., and, more recently, retrospective series have been reported [56, 57]. The pro-cedure was reported to have a high rate of technical success (99.5%) and a low complication rate (1.5%) [57]. Presently, there is no consensus on which type of stent should be used, and opera-tors often use peripheral stents (e.g., Wallstent [Boston Scientific], Acculink [Abbott Vascular], Precise [Cordis], Protégé [Medtronic], and Zilver [Cook Medical]). Improvement of the pressure gradi-ent within the sinuses is usually observed immediately during post-stent deployment measurements, and symptoms improve over a few days and weeks. According to a recent meta-analysis, VSS results in improvement of headache, papilledema, and tinni-tus in 79.6%, 93.7%, and 90.3% of patients, respectively [58]. Although these results are promising, de novo stenosis can recur within the stented portion of the sinus or adjacent to the stent in up to 16% of patients, often accompanied by a recurrent increased pressure gradient and symptoms requiring retreatment [58]. Another interesting use of VSS was recently reported in a more acute setting for a few patients who presented with fulminant visual deficits, with good results and preventing permanent visual loss [59–61].

Therefore, VSS has led to some additional clarity of the inciting and persistent mechanisms of IIH. It is expected that newer stents optimized for this use will become available in the near future, and treatment indications with more solid recommendations will be delineated.

Endovascular Management of Hydrocephalus

In addition to recent advancements in the treatment of IIH and venous pathologies of the brain, there are exciting new technologies under development to address hydrocephalus through endovascular means. One such technological innovation is the eShunt System (CereVasc, LLC), which is an endovascular transluminal catheter-deployed shunt designed to be implanted into the inferior petrosal sinus [62]. This biomimetic transluminal shunt is designed to serve in an analogous function to the arachnoid granulations of the brain, providing a direct CSF-to-venous outflow tract without the intervening need for a subcutaneous catheter or an implantable mechanical valve [62]. Surgically implanted ventricular CSF shunts are often plagued by mechanical issues or infection, especially in the immediate postimplantation period, requiring revision surgery. Ventricular shunts have been found to have a 15–25% 30-day failure rate, with 1-year failure rates of up to 28% [63, 64]. This high rate of failure is associated with vastly increased costs of care and contributes to a cumulative yearly cost of more than $1 billion in the USA alone [65]. The need for repeat revisions, extended hospital stays, and potential life-threatening consequences of shunt failure is burdensome to patients, their families, providers, and the hospital system. A meaningful, minimally invasive treatment for hydrocephalus could therefore address an area of critical need and improve patient recovery and outcomes. Presently, a pilot clinical trial is underway in Argentina (ETCHES I), and initial use of the eShunt System in patients with communicating hydrocephalus has been successfully reported [66]. Although this technology provides an exciting potential treatment opportunity for a particularly troublesome thorn in the neurosurgeon's side, the onus will be on endovascular surgeons to ensure the safety and efficacy if it is to be implemented in clinical practice.

Stentrodes for Endovascular Neuromodulation

Brain-computer interfaces (BCI) offer great potential in restoring voluntary motor activity secondary to motor paralysis from a number of conditions that affect the brain, spinal cord, and peripheral nerves [67–71]. Patients who suffer from impaired motor functioning struggle with their activities of daily living (ADL) [70]. An implantable neuroprosthesis serves as a conduit for communication between the electrical activity of the motor cortex and the computer interface so that day-to-day activities such as communication, financial management, and online shopping can be performed in a relatively seamless manner [72–75].

A handful of early feasibility studies have shown promising results with the use of the implantable Stentrode BCI (Synchron) in patients with varying degrees and types of motor paralysis [75–78]. Most recently, Oxley et al. described the first in-human experience using a minimally invasive, endovascularly delivered, wireless Stentrode BCI in two patients with complete motor paralysis secondary to amyotrophic lateral sclerosis [75]. The Stentrode BCI, a self-expandable, monolithic thin-film stent electrode array, is implanted endovascularly in the superior sagittal sinus (Fig. 1.4), adjacent to the precentral motor gyrus, which was mapped presurgically using MRI [75]. Sixteen sensors are positioned circumferentially on the nitinol scaffold in the superior sagittal sinus and connected to a transvascular lead that is inserted

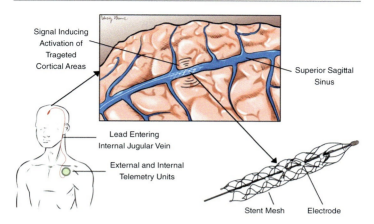

Fig. 1.4 Illustration showing neuromodulation with a Stentrode (Synchron). An internal telemetry unit implanted within the chest muscles receives signal from an external telemetry unit. The signal is transduced through the lead, which then enters venous circulation through the internal jugular vein and goes up to the superior sagittal sinus, where the Stentrode induces activation of targeted cortical areas

into an internal telemetry unit placed within the subclavicular space [75]. An external telemetry unit conductively powers the internal telemetry unit, receiving an electrocorticography signal through infrared light transmission [75]. The signal is then transmitted to the computer tablet through a signal control unit, which translates the signal into multiple-click actions through a custom decoder [75]. This multiple command control is combined with eye tracking to perform computer operations. Postprocedure, participants are engaged in motor mapping tasks, guiding the on-screen pointers. This study showed very encouraging results in terms of click selection accuracy for both patients (92.6% and 93.2%, respectively) and successful completion of several ADL tasks including messaging, independently managing finances, and online shopping [75]. Another study by Chen et al. demonstrated the use of a similar submillimetric, wireless, and battery-free implant in the peripheral nervous system [77]. A digitally programmable system-on-a-chip implantable device is delivered endovascularly and placed adjacent to the sciatic nerve, allowing for wireless stimulation of the nerves [77].

Endovascular and minimally invasive delivery and implantation of the sophisticated Stentrode BCI in the brain is an important step forward and a major improvement when compared to the landmark fully implantable BCI study by Vansteensel et al. in which a burr-hole craniotomy was required to place the devices and the result of achieving a single binary click was modest [78]. With the advent and present application of the Stentrode BCI, less supervised training, greater range of applicability, and quicker recovery postprocedure offer promise for not only advanced patient care but also expanding indications for endovascular neurosurgery.

Conclusions

The future of neurointervention is bright and ever expanding. However, innovation and increase in demand generate concerns, as in any other burgeoning field. Operators must be up to date with novel treatment alternatives; trainees are exposed to larger skill sets to be learned and mastered; and efforts must be joined to improve not only the distribution and reach of endovascular modalities but also the quality of care being delivered. Multidisciplinary collaborations between neurointervention and other fields will likely expand the frontiers of neuroendovascular therapies to conditions previously managed in completely different ways.

Acknowledgments   We thank Paul H. Dressel BFA for formatting the illustrations and Debra J Zimmer for editorial support.

Disclosure of Relationships/Potential Conflicts of Interest   *WM-D, AM, WIK*—None

AHS—Consulting fees: Amnis Therapeutics, Apellis Pharmaceuticals, Inc., Boston Scientific, Canon Medical Systems USA, Inc., Cardinal Health 200, LLC, Cerebrotech Medical Systems, Inc., Cerenovus, Cerevatech Medical, Inc., Cordis, Corindus, Inc., Endostream Medical, Ltd., Imperative Care,

InspireMD, Ltd., Integra, IRRAS AB, Medtronic, MicroVention, Minnetronix Neuro, Inc., Peijia Medical, Penumbra, Q'Apel Medical, Inc., Rapid Medical, Serenity Medical, Inc., Silk Road Medical, StimMed, LLC, Stryker Neurovascular, Three Rivers Medical, Inc., VasSol, Viz.ai, Inc. Leadership or fiduciary role in other board, society, committee, or advocacy group: Secretary, Board of the Society of NeuroInterventional Surgery 2020–2021; Chair, Cerebrovascular Section of the AANS/CNS 2020–2021. Stock or stock options: Adona Medical, Inc., Amnis Therapeutics, Bend, IT Technologies, Ltd., BlinkTBI, Inc., Cerebrotech Medical Systems, Inc., Cerevatech Medical, Inc., Cognition Medical, CVAID Ltd., E8, Inc., Endostream Medical, Ltd., Galaxy Therapeutics, Inc., Imperative; Care, Inc., InspireMD, Ltd., Instylla, Inc., International Medical Distribution Partners, Launch NY, Inc.; Neurolutions, Inc., NeuroRadial Technologies, Inc., NeuroTechnology Investors, Neurovascular Diagnostics, Inc., Peijia; Medical, PerFlow Medical, Ltd., Q'Apel Medical, Inc., QAS.ai, Inc., Radical Catheter Technologies, Inc., Rebound Therapeutics Corp. (purchased 2019 by Integra Lifesciences, Corp), Rist Neurovascular, Inc. (purchased 2020 by Medtronic), Sense Diagnostics, Inc., Serenity Medical, Inc., Silk Road Medical, Sim & Cure, SongBird Therapy, Spinnaker Medical, Inc., StimMed, LLC, Synchron, Inc., Three Rivers Medical, Inc., Truvic Medical, Inc., Tulavi Therapeutics, Inc., Vastrax, LLC, VICIS, Inc., Viseon, Inc. Other financial or nonfinancial interests: National PI/Steering Committees: Cerenovus EXCELLENT and ARISE II Trial; Medtronic SWIFT PRIME, VANTAGE, EMBOLISE, and SWIFT DIRECT Trials; MicroVention FRED Trial & CONFIDENCE Study; MUSC POSITIVE Trial; Penumbra 3D Separator Trial, COMPASS Trial, INVEST Trial, and MIVI neuroscience EVAQ Trial; Rapid Medical SUCCESS Trial; InspireMD C-GUARDIANS IDE Pivotal Trial.

EIL—Shareholder/Ownership Interest: NeXtGen Biologics, RAPID Medical, Claret Medical, Cognition Medical, Imperative Care, Rebound Therapeutics, StimMed, Three Rivers Medical; Patent: Bone Scalpel; Honorarium for Training & Lectures: Medtronic, Penumbra, MicroVention, Integra, Consultant: Clarion, GLG Consulting, Guidepoint Global, Imperative Care, Medtronic, StimMed, Misionix, Mosaic; Chief Medical Officer: Haniva Technology; National PI: Medtronic—Steering Committees for SWIFT Prime and SWIFT Direct Trials; Site PI Study: MicroVention (CONFIDENCE Study), Medtronic (STRATIS Study-Sub 1); Advisory Board: Stryker (AIS Clinical Advisory Board), NeXtGen Biologics, MEDX, Cognition Medical; Endostream Medical, IRRAS AB (Consultant/Advisory Board), Medical Legal Review: renders medical/legal opinions as an expert witness; Leadership or fiduciary roles in other board society, committee, or advocacy group, paid and unpaid: CNS, ABNS, UBNS.

References

1. Smith WS, Furlan AJ. Brief history of endovascular acute Ischemic stroke treatment. Stroke. 2016;47(2):e23–6.
2. Mocco J, Hanel RA, Sharma J, et al. Use of a vascular reconstruction device to salvage acute ischemic occlusions refractory to traditional endovascular recanalization methods. J Neurosurg. 2010;112(3):557–62.
3. Goyal M, Menon BK, van Zwam WH, et al. Endovascular thrombectomy after large-vessel ischaemic stroke: a meta-analysis of individual patient data from five randomised trials. Lancet. 2016;387(10029):1723–31.
4. Albers GW, Marks MP, Kemp S, et al. Thrombectomy for stroke at 6 to 16 hours with selection by perfusion imaging. N Engl J Med. 2018;378(8):708–18.
5. Nogueira RG, Jadhav AP, Haussen DC, et al. Thrombectomy 6 to 24 hours after stroke with a mismatch between deficit and infarct. N Engl J Med. 2018;378(1):11–21.
6. Mokin M, Levy EI, Saver JL, et al. Predictive value of RAPID assessed perfusion thresholds on final infarct volume in SWIFT PRIME (Solitaire with the intention for Thrombectomy as primary endovascular treatment). Stroke. 2017;48(4):932–8.
7. Turk AS 3rd, Siddiqui A, Fifi JT, et al. Aspiration thrombectomy versus stent retriever thrombectomy as first-line approach for large vessel occlusion (COMPASS): a multicentre, randomised, open label, blinded outcome, non-inferiority trial. Lancet. 2019;393(10175):998–1008.
8. Cortez GM, Turner RD, Monteiro A, et al. Walrus large bore guide catheter impact on recanalization first pass effect and outcomes: the WICkED study. J Neurointerv Surg. 2022;14(3):280–5.
9. Siddiqui AH, Waqas M, Neumaier J, et al. Radial first or patient first: a case series and meta-analysis of transradial versus transfemoral access for acute ischemic stroke intervention. J Neurointerv Surg. 2021;13(8):687–92.
10. Dossani RH, Waqas M, Rai HH, et al. Use of Walrus balloon-guide catheter through sheathless radial approach for mechanical thrombectomy of right middle cerebral artery occlusion. J Neurointerv Surg. 2022;14(5):neurintsurg-2021-017985.
11. Goyal M, Kappelhof M, Ospel JM, Bala F. Balloon guide catheters: use, reject, or randomize? Neuroradiology. 2021;63(8):1179–83.
12. Dossani RH, Waqas M, Monteiro A, et al. Use of a sheathless 8-French balloon guide catheter (Walrus) through the radial artery for mechanical thrombectomy: technique and case series. J Neurointerv Surg. 2022;14(5):neurintsurg-2021-017868.
13. Zaidat OO, Mueller-Kronast NH, Hassan AE, et al. Impact of balloon guide catheter use on clinical and angiographic outcomes in the STRATIS stroke Thrombectomy registry. Stroke. 2019;50(3):697–704.

14. Lin CH, Saver JL, Ovbiagele B, Huang WY, Lee M. Endovascular thrombectomy without versus with intravenous thrombolysis in acute ischemic stroke: a non-inferiority meta-analysis of randomized clinical trials. J Neurointerv Surg. 2022;14(3):227–32.
15. Zi W, Qiu Z, Li F, et al. Effect of endovascular treatment alone vs Intravenous Alteplase Plus endovascular treatment on functional independence in patients with acute ischemic stroke: the DEVT randomized clinical trial. JAMA. 2021;325(3):234–43.
16. Yang P, Zhang Y, Zhang L, et al. Endovascular Thrombectomy with or without intravenous Alteplase in acute stroke. N Engl J Med. 2020;382(21):1981–93.
17. Suzuki K, Matsumaru Y, Takeuchi M, et al. Effect of mechanical Thrombectomy without vs with intravenous thrombolysis on functional outcome among patients with acute ischemic stroke: the SKIP randomized clinical trial. JAMA. 2021;325(3):244–53.
18. Horowitz MB, Levy E, Kassam A, Purdy PD. Endovascular therapy for intracranial aneurysms: a historical and present status review. Surg Neurol. 2002;57(3):147–158; discussion 158–149.
19. Jahshan S, Abla AA, Natarajan SK, et al. Results of stent-assisted vs non-stent-assisted endovascular therapies in 489 cerebral aneurysms: single-center experience. Neurosurgery. 2013;72(2):232–9.
20. Monteiro A, Cortez GM, Aghaebrahim A, Sauvageau E, Hanel RA. Low-profile visualized intraluminal support Jr Braided Stent versus Atlas self-expandable stent for treatment of intracranial Aneurysms: a single center experience. Neurosurgery. 2021;88(2):E170–e178.
21. Hanel RA, Kallmes DF, Lopes DK, et al. Prospective study on embolization of intracranial aneurysms with the pipeline device: the PREMIER study 1 year results. J Neurointerv Surg. 2020;12(1):62–6.
22. Natarajan SK, Lin N, Sonig A, et al. The safety of Pipeline flow diversion in fusiform vertebrobasilar aneurysms: a consecutive case series with longer-term follow-up from a single US center. J Neurosurg. 2016;125(1):111–9.
23. Cappuzzo JM, Monteiro A, Taylor MN, et al. First U.S. experience using the Pipeline Flex Embolization device with Shield technology for treatment of intracranial aneurysms. World Neurosurg. 2022;159:e184–91.
24. Oliver AA, Carlson KD, Bilgin C, et al. Bioresorbable flow diverters for the treatment of intracranial aneurysms: review of current literature and future directions. J NeuroInterven Surg. 2022;15:178.
25. Monteiro A, Lazar AL, Waqas M, et al. Treatment of ruptured intracranial aneurysms with the Woven EndoBridge device: a systematic review. J Neurointerv Surg. 2022;14(4):366–70.
26. Lim J, Vakharia K, Waqas M, et al. Comaneci device for temporary coiling assistance for treatment of wide-necked Aneurysms: initial case series and systematic literature review. World Neurosurg. 2021;149:e85–91.

27. Waqas M, Monteiro A, Cappuzzo JM, Tutino VM, Levy EI. Evolution of the patient-first approach: a dual-trained, single-neurosurgeon experience with 2002 consecutive intracranial aneurysm treatments. J Neurosurg. 2022;137:1–7.

28. Sarraj A, Savitz S, Pujara D, et al. Endovascular Thrombectomy for acute Ischemic strokes: current US Access Paradigms and optimization methodology. Stroke. 2020;51(4):1207–17.

29. Aldstadt J, Waqas M, Yasumiishi M, et al. Mapping access to endovascular stroke care in the USA and implications for transport models. J Neurointerv Surg. 2022;14(1):neurintsurg-2020-016942.

30. Linfante I, Nogueira RG, Zaidat OO, et al. A joint statement from the Neurointerventional Societies: our position on operator experience and training for stroke thrombectomy. J Neurointerv Surg. 2019;11(6):533–4.

31. Kim BM, Baek JH, Heo JH, Kim DJ, Nam HS, Kim YD. Effect of cumulative case volume on procedural and clinical outcomes in endovascular Thrombectomy. Stroke. 2019;50(5):1178–83.

32. Stein LK, Mocco J, Fifi J, Jette N, Tuhrim S, Dhamoon MS. Correlations between physician and hospital stroke Thrombectomy volumes and outcomes: a nationwide analysis. Stroke. 2021;52(9):2858–65.

33. Waqas M, Tutino VM, Cappuzzo JM, et al. Stroke thrombectomy volume, rather than stroke center accreditation status of hospitals, is associated with mortality and discharge disposition. J Neurointerv Surg. 2022;15:209.

34. Levy EI, Boulos AS, Fessler RD, et al. Transradial cerebral angiography: an alternative route. Neurosurgery. 2002;51(2):335–340; discussion 340–332.

35. Waqas M, Vakharia K, Dossani RH, et al. Transradial access for flow diversion of intracranial aneurysms: case series. Interv Neuroradiol. 2021;27(1):68–74.

36. Waqas M, Monteiro A, Baig AA, et al. Rist Guide Catheter for endovascular procedures: initial case series from a single center. Interv Neuroradiol. 2022;29:108. https://doi.org/10.1177/15910199221074884.

37. Tso MK, Rajah GB, Dossani RH, et al. Learning curves for transradial access versus transfemoral access in diagnostic cerebral angiography: a case series. J Neurointerv Surg. 2022;14(2):174–8.

38. Monteiro A, Cappuzzo JM, Aguirre AO, et al. Transradial versus Transfemoral approach for Neuroendovascular procedures: a survey of patient preferences and perspectives, vol. 2022. World Neurosurg; 2022. p. e623.

39. Joshi KC, Beer-Furlan A, Crowley RW, Chen M, Munich SA. Transradial approach for neurointerventions: a systematic review of the literature. J Neurointerv Surg. 2020;12(9):886–92.

40. Mendes Pereira V, Cancelliere NM, Nicholson P, et al. First-in-human, robotic-assisted neuroendovascular intervention. J Neurointerv Surg. 2020;12(4):338–40.

41. Crinnion W, Jackson B, Sood A, et al. Robotics in neurointerventional surgery: a systematic review of the literature. J Neurointerv Surg. 2022;14(6):539–45.
42. Farb RI, Nicholson PJ, Peng PW, et al. Spontaneous intracranial hypotension: a systematic imaging approach for CSF leak localization and management based on MRI and digital subtraction myelography. AJNR Am J Neuroradiol. 2019;40(4):745–53.
43. Brinjikji W, Savastano LE, Atkinson JLD, Garza I, Farb R, Cutsforth-Gregory JK. A novel endovascular therapy for CSF hypotension secondary to CSF-Venous Fistulas. AJNR Am J Neuroradiol. 2021;42(5):882–7.
44. Brinjikji W, Garza I, Whealy M, et al. Clinical and imaging outcomes of cerebrospinal fluid-venous fistula embolization. J Neurointerv Surg. 2022;14:953.
45. Shlobin NA, Shah VN, Chin CT, Dillon WP, Tan LA. Cerebrospinal Fluid-Venous Fistulas: a systematic review and examination of individual patient data. Neurosurgery. 2021;88(5):931–41.
46. Borg N, Oushy S, Savastano L, Brinjikji W. Transvenous embolization of a cerebrospinal fluid-venous fistula for the treatment of spontaneous intracranial hypotension. J Neurointerv Surg. 2021;14:948.
47. Degnan AJ, Levy LM. Pseudotumor cerebri: brief review of clinical syndrome and imaging findings. AJNR Am J Neuroradiol. 2011;32(11):1986–93.
48. Levitt MR, Hlubek RJ, Moon K, et al. Incidence and predictors of dural venous sinus pressure gradient in idiopathic intracranial hypertension and non-idiopathic intracranial hypertension headache patients: results from 164 cerebral venograms. J Neurosurg. 2017;126(2):347–53.
49. Baryshnik DB, Farb RI. Changes in the appearance of venous sinuses after treatment of disordered intracranial pressure. Neurology. 2004;62(8):1445–6.
50. Horev A, Hallevy H, Plakht Y, Shorer Z, Wirguin I, Shelef I. Changes in cerebral venous sinuses diameter after lumbar puncture in idiopathic intracranial hypertension: a prospective MRI study. J Neuroimaging. 2013;23(3):375–8.
51. Lee SW, Gates P, Morris P, Whan A, Riddington L. Idiopathic intracranial hypertension; immediate resolution of venous sinus "obstruction" after reducing cerebrospinal fluid pressure to<10cmH(2)O. J Clin Neurosci. 2009;16(12):1690–2.
52. Stienen A, Weinzierl M, Ludolph A, Tibussek D, Häusler M. Obstruction of cerebral venous sinus secondary to idiopathic intracranial hypertension. Eur J Neurol. 2008;15(12):1416–8.
53. Buell TJ, Raper DMS, Pomeraniec IJ, et al. Transient resolution of venous sinus stenosis after high-volume lumbar puncture in a patient with idiopathic intracranial hypertension. J Neurosurg. 2018;129(1):153–6.
54. Fargen KM. A unifying theory explaining venous sinus stenosis and recurrent stenosis following venous sinus stenting in patients with idiopathic intracranial hypertension. J Neurointerv Surg. 2021;13(7):587–92.

55. Cappuzzo JM, Hess RM, Morrison JF, et al. Transverse venous stenting for the treatment of idiopathic intracranial hypertension, or pseudotumor cerebri. Neurosurg Focus. 2018;45(1):E11.

56. Higgins JN, Owler BK, Cousins C, Pickard JD. Venous sinus stenting for refractory benign intracranial hypertension. Lancet. 2002;359(9302):228–30.

57. Leishangthem L, SirDeshpande P, Dua D, Satti SR. Dural venous sinus stenting for idiopathic intracranial hypertension: an updated review. J Neuroradiol. 2019;46(2):148–54.

58. Saber H, Lewis W, Sadeghi M, Rajah G, Narayanan S. Stent survival and stent-adjacent stenosis rates following Venous Sinus stenting for idiopathic intracranial hypertension: a systematic review and meta-analysis. Interv Neurol. 2018;7(6):490–500.

59. Elder BD, Goodwin CR, Kosztowski TA, et al. Venous sinus stenting is a valuable treatment for fulminant idiopathic intracranial hypertension. J Clin Neurosci. 2015;22(4):685–9.

60. Monteiro A, Fritz AG, Cappuzzo JM, Waqas M, Levy EI, Siddiqui AH. Venous sinus stenting for the treatment of acute blindness in a patient with idiopathic intracranial hypertension. Interv Neuroradiol. 2022;29:605. https://doi.org/10.1177/15910199221095973.

61. Zehri AH, Lee KE, Kartchner J, et al. Efficacy of dural venous sinus stenting in treating idiopathic intracranial hypertension with acute vision loss. Neuroradiol J. 2022;35(1):86–93.

62. Heilman CB, Basil GW, Beneduce BM, Malek AM. Anatomical characterization of the inferior petrosal sinus and adjacent cerebellopontine angle cistern for development of an endovascular transdural cerebrospinal fluid shunt. J Neurointerv Surg. 2019;11(6):598–602.

63. Al-Tamimi YZ, Sinha P, Chumas PD, et al. Ventriculoperitoneal shunt 30-day failure rate: a retrospective international cohort study. Neurosurgery. 2014;74(1):29–34.

64. Anderson IA, Saukila LF, Robins JMW, et al. Factors associated with 30-day ventriculoperitoneal shunt failure in pediatric and adult patients. J Neurosurg. 2018;130(1):145–53.

65. Patwardhan RV, Nanda A. Implanted ventricular shunts in the United States: the billion-dollar-a-year cost of hydrocephalus treatment. Neurosurgery. 2005;56(1):139–144; discussion 144–135.

66. Lylyk P, Lylyk I, Bleise C, et al. LB-001 First in-human treatment of communicating hydrocephalus using the CereVasc eShunt™ miniature biomimetic endovascular CSF shunt. J NeuroIntervent Surg. 2021;13(Suppl 1):A145.

67. Graham DM. Minimally invasive brain recordings with a 'stentrode'. Lab Anim (NY). 2016;45(5):158.

68. Opie NL, van der Nagel NR, John SE, et al. Micro-CT and histological evaluation of an neural interface implanted within a blood vessel. IEEE Trans Biomed Eng. 2017;64(4):928–34.

69. Godil A, Hafiz MY, Shoaib M. Stentrode - on way to revolutionize neuro-sciences. J Pak Med Assoc. 2016;66(8):1047.
70. Rajah G, Saber H, Singh R, Rangel-Castilla L. Endovascular delivery of leads and stentrodes and their applications to deep brain stimulation and neuromodulation: a review. Neurosurg Focus. 2018;45(2):E19.
71. Raza SA, Opie NL, Morokoff A, Sharma RP, Mitchell PJ, Oxley TJ. Endovascular neuromodulation: safety profile and future directions. Front Neurol. 2020;11:351.
72. Gerboni G, John SE, Ronayne SM, et al. Cortical brain stimulation with endovascular electrodes. Annu Int Conf IEEE Eng Med Biol Soc. 2018;2018:3088–91.
73. Obidin N, Tasnim F, Dagdeviren C. The future of neuroimplantable devices: a materials science and regulatory perspective. Adv Mater. 2020;32(15):e1901482.
74. John SE, Grayden DB, Yanagisawa T. The future potential of the Stentrode. Expert Rev Med Devices. 2019;16(10):841–3.
75. Oxley TJ, Yoo PE, Rind GS, et al. Motor neuroprosthesis implanted with neurointerventional surgery improves capacity for activities of daily living tasks in severe paralysis: first in-human experience. J Neurointerv Surg. 2021;13(2):102–8.
76. Han JJ. Synchron receives FDA approval to begin early feasibility study of their endovascular, brain-computer interface device. Artif Organs. 2021;45(10):1134–5.
77. Chen JC, Kan P, Yu Z, et al. A wireless millimetric magnetoelectric implant for the endovascular stimulation of peripheral nerves. Nat Biomed Eng. 2022;6:706.
78. Vansteensel MJ, Pels EGM, Bleichner MG, et al. Fully implanted brain-computer interface in a locked-in patient with ALS. N Engl J Med. 2016;375(21):2060–6.

Minimally Invasive Intracerebral Hemorrhage Removal

2

Jack Jestus, Demi Dawkins,
Kenneth Moore, Adam Arthur,
and Christopher Nickele

Introduction

Spontaneous intracerebral hemorrhage (ICH) represents up to 20% of all strokes and remains one of the most dangerous stroke subsets, with high morbidity and mortality rates. Despite its severity, there is still no definitive treatment for this disease [1]. Care can range from medical management to surgical evacuation or decompression. The goal of surgery is generally to treat mass effect and reduce elevated intracranial pressure (ICP) in addition to preventing secondary neurological injury related to cerebral edema [1, 2]. Applying the advancements in minimally invasive

J. Jestus
Neurosurgery, University of Tennessee Health Science Center, Memphis, TN, USA

D. Dawkins
Neurosurgery, Semmes Murphey Clinic, Memphis, TN, United States

K. Moore · A. Arthur, · C. Nickele (✉)
Neurosurgery, University of Tennessee Health Science Center, Memphis, TN, USA

Neurosurgery, Semmes Murphey Clinic, Memphis, TN, United States
e-mail: cnickele@semmes-murphey.com

© The Author(s), under exclusive license to Springer Nature Switzerland AG 2025
E. Veznedaroglu (ed.), *Advanced Technologies in Vascular Neurosurgery*, https://doi.org/10.1007/978-3-031-67492-1_2

27

surgery (MIS) to surgical treatment of ICH potentially allows for safer hematoma evacuation with less risk of injury to the adjacent normal brain parenchyma.

This chapter reviews the various treatment options for MIS ICH evacuation and the associated literature. Table 2.1 illustrates a summary of some of the techniques discussed in this review and their respective study results (Table 2.1) [1].

STICH Trial

The STICH (Surgical Trial in Intracerebral Hemorrhage) trials were some of the first large-scale clinical trials to evaluate the benefits of surgical intervention with craniotomy and hematoma evacuation compared to nonsurgical treatment for ICH [3, 4]. For STICH I, 1033 patients with supratentorial ICH were randomized to early surgery or initial conservative medical management. Patients randomized to medical management could undergo surgery if needed after randomization, but results were analyzed on intention-to-treat basis. Results were based on the Glasgow Outcome Scale at a 6-month follow-up. There was not a significant difference in neurological function at 6 months between the early intervention group and the initial medical therapy group. While this trial seems to suggest that early surgical intervention has no effect on the neurological outcome of the patient, subgroup analysis did note improved outcomes when the hematoma is more superficial [3]. STICH II then sought to demonstrate the benefit of hematoma evacuation for hematomas on the cortical surface, but ultimately it failed [4].

There are many possible reasons why these trials likely did not show any positive benefit to using surgical treatment of ICH. One reason is the rate of crossover from medical management to surgery in STICH I, which was 140 out of 530 patients (26%) randomized to initial medical management. STICH II had 62 patients of 292 crossover from initial medical management to surgery (21%). Another reason is the surgical technique utilized in the study. New, less invasive surgical techniques continue to be considered to further elucidate the potential benefit of surgery on ICH

Table 2.1 Summary of research studies evaluated

Study	Completed or ongoing	MIS technique	Dates of enrollment	Location	Number of subjects	Results[a]
Wang et al. [8]	Completed	Craniopuncture	January 2003 to June 2004	42 centers in China	195 craniopuncture vs 182 conservative medical management	*Mortality:* 6.7% vs 8.8% ($p = 0.44$) at 90 days *Functional status:* Barthel Index (BI) increase at 90 days ($x^2 = 23.13$, $p = 0.0001$) *Rebleeding:* 9.7% vs 5.0%, $p = 0.08$
Sun et al. [7]	Completed	Craniopuncture	January 2003 to July 2005	22 centers in China	159 craniopuncture with urokinase vs 145 craniotomy	*Mortality:* 14.5% vs 25.0% ($p = 0.02$) at 90 days *Functional status:* no difference in BI at 90 days ($x^2 = 4.166$, $p = 0.38$) *Rebleeding:* 8.8% vs 21.4%, $p = 0.002$
Zhou et al. [9]	Completed	Craniopuncture	2005–2008	China	90 craniopuncture vs 78 craniotomy	*Mortality:* 18.9% vs 24.4% ($p = 0.39$) at 365 days *Functional status:* BI = 79.5 vs 62 ($p = 0.01$) at 365 days *Rebleeding:* 10.0% vs 15.4%, $p = 0.29$

(continued)

Table 2.1 (continued)

Study	Completed or ongoing	MIS technique	Dates of enrollment	Location	Number of subjects	Results[a]
Stereotactic Treatment of Intracerebral Hematoma by Means of a Plasminogen Activator (SICHPA)	Completed	Stereotactic evacuation with thrombolysis	March 1996 to May 1999	13 centers in the Netherlands	36 surgical vs 35 nonsurgical	*Mortality:* 56% vs 59% ($p = 0.78$) at 180 days *Functional status:* no difference in likelihood of mRS > 4 (OR = 0.52, $p = 0.38$) *Rebleeding:* 0% vs 22%, $p = 0.006$
Minimally Invasive Surgery Plus Rt-PA for ICH Evacuation Phase 3 (MISTIE 3)	Completed	Stereotactic evacuation with thrombolysis	December 2013 to August 2017	84 centers: Australia, Canada, China, Germany, Hungary, Israel, Spain, UK, and USA	255 MISTIE vs 251 standard medical care	*Mortality:* 19% vs 26% ($p = 0.04$) at 365 days *Functional status:* no difference in mRS < 4 at 365 days (45% vs 41%, $p = 0.33$) *Rebleeding:* 2% vs 1%, $p = 0.32$

					Expected enrollment: 300	Study ongoing—N/A
Early Minimally Invasive Removal of Intracerebral Hemorrhage (ENRICH)	Ongoing	Endoport-mediated evacuation	December 2016 to December 2021	36 centers in the USA	Expected enrollment: 300	Study ongoing—N/A
Auer et al. [18]	Completed	Endoscope-assisted evacuation	June 1983 to August 1986	Austria	50 endoscope vs 50 medical management	*Mortality:* 42% vs 70% ($p < 0.01$) at 180 days *Functional status:* significant difference in "minimal neurologic deficit" at 180 days (40% vs 25%, $p < 0.05$) *Rebleeding:* 4% vs 30%, $p < 0.05$
Intraoperative Stereotactic Computed Tomography-Guided Endoscopic Surgery (ICES)	Completed	Endoscope-assisted evacuation	August 2005 to August 2012	29 centers: Canada, Germany, USA, and UK	14 surgical vs four medical management	*Mortality:* 0% vs 7.1% ($p = 0.68$) *Functional status:* no difference in mRS < 4 at 180 days (42% vs 24%, $p = 0.19$) *Rebleeding:* no rebleeding in either group

(continued)

Table 2.1 (continued)

Study	Completed or ongoing	MIS technique	Dates of enrollment	Location	Number of subjects	Results[a]
Spiotta et al. [28]	Completed	Adjunctive aspiration device	May 2014 to September 2014	Four centers: USA	29 Apollo	*Mortality:* 13.8% (*n* = 4) *Mean ICH volume reduction:* 54.1 ± 39.1%, *p* < 0.001
Goyal et al. [29]	Completed	Adjunctive aspiration device	July 2014 to December 2017	One center: USA	18 surgical vs 54 medical management	*Mortality:* 28% vs 56%, *p* = 0.041 *Functional status:* no difference in mRS at discharge or 3 months (*p* = 0.407 and 0.521, respectively) *Median ICH volume at 24 hours:* 40 cm³ vs 15 cm³, *p* < 0.001
Minimally Invasive Endoscopic Surgery with Apollo in Patients with Brain Hemorrhage (INVEST)	Ongoing	Adjunctive aspiration device (Apollo)	June 2017 to June 2021	Seven centers in USA	Estimated enrollment: 50	Study ongoing—N/A

Artemis in the Removal of Intracerebral Hemorrhage (MIND)	Ongoing	Adjunctive aspiration device (Artemis)	February 2018 to July 2024	20 locations in Germany and USA	Estimated enrollment: 500	Study ongoing—N/A
Dutch Intracerebral Hemorrhage Surgery Trial (DIST)	Ongoing	Adjunctive aspiration device (Artemis)	November 2018–present	Ten centers in the Netherlands	Estimated enrollment: 600	Study ongoing—N/A
Minimally Invasive Intracerebral Hemorrhage Evacuation (MIRROR)	Ongoing	Surgiscope	October 2020 to October 2028	Two centers in the USA	Estimated enrollment: 500	Study ongoing—N/A

(continued)

Table 2.1 (continued)

Study	Completed or ongoing	MIS technique	Dates of enrollment	Location	Number of subjects	Results[a]
Ultra-Early, Minimally Invasive Intracerebral Hemorrhage Evacuation Versus Standard Treatment (EVACUATE)	Ongoing	Surgiscope	September 2020 to December 2025	Two centers in Australia	Estimated enrollment: 240	Study ongoing—N/A
Newell et al. [30]	Completed	Sonothrombolysis	November 2008 to July 2009	One center: USA	Nine surgical	*Mortality:* 11% (*n* = 1) *Functional status:* NIH Stroke Scale decreased from 17.6 to 8.5 *Mean volume reduction at 24 hours:* 59 ± 5% for ICH; 45.1 ± 13% for IVH

[a]Results for each category correspond respectively to their distinguished order in the "Number of subjects" column

treatment. It is hypothesized that MIS could reduce the damage to surrounding brain tissue that likely occurred in this study population.

Animal Models of MIS for ICH Evacuation

Multiple animal models of ICH and minimally invasive evacuation have been developed which demonstrate decreased blood-brain barrier (BBB) permeability and other markers of cerebral tissue damage in animals that undergo minimally invasive evacuation of induced ICH when compared to control models that do not undergo evacuation of an induced hemorrhage [2, 5]. The authors of these studies suggest that reduction in these factors may translate to decreased secondary cerebral edema and thus decreased secondary neuronal injury. Studies such as these form the basis of interest in minimally invasive surgical ICH evacuation.

Meta-Analysis of MIS Trials

Scaggiante et al. conducted a meta-analysis of 2152 patients enrolled in 15 randomized clinical trials for supratentorial spontaneous ICH treatment [6]. This study attempted to determine the benefits of MIS on ICH in addition to the effects of quick treatment (<24 hours post-ictus) on neurological outcome. This study was able to demonstrate a decrease in "moderate-to-severe" functional impairment and mortality at long-term follow-up compared to conventional treatment. As well, they demonstrated that patients who received ICH evacuation within 24 hours (or within 72 hours) of ictus were more likely to achieve functional independence when compared to patients treated outside of that timeframe. The results of this study help strengthen the case for the further development of MIS-ICH techniques in an attempt to discover an effective treatment for this disease.

Review of MIS Techniques

Craniopuncture

Craniopuncture remains the standard of care for ICH treatment in China, although no large-scale clinical trials have taken place in Europe or the USA. With this technique, a puncture needle is drilled through the skull to the hematoma. The needle is then attached to the skull, and hematoma evacuation is performed with the assistance of a thrombolytic agent. The cannula is left in place, and a thrombolytic agent is delivered to the hematoma every 6–12 hours. The needle remains in situ for 3–5 days [1].

Three major studies based in China have taken place to evaluate the effects of craniopuncture, and all three demonstrate some evidence of benefit compared to nonsurgical treatment [7–9]. Wang et al. reported a multicenter randomized controlled trial comparing craniopuncture to medical management for treatment of basal ganglia hemorrhages in 377 patients. This demonstrated significant early improvement in neurological function (at 2 weeks) and significantly lower proportion of patients with modified Rankin Scale (mRS) >2 at 3 months but with no significant difference in mortality rates [8]. Sun et al. conducted a multicenter randomized controlled trial of 304 patients comparing craniopuncture to small craniotomy for evacuation of basal ganglia hemorrhages. This study demonstrated no difference in neurological function or mRS between the two groups, but there was a significant decrease in mortality at 90 days and rebleeding after surgery in the craniopuncture group [7]. Finally, Zhou et al. conducted a single center randomized controlled trial of 168 patients with basal ganglia or lobar hemorrhages comparing craniopuncture to craniotomy for hematoma evacuation. Their study demonstrated no significant difference in rebleed rate or mortality but did note significant improvement in mRS at 1 year [9]. This group of studies inconsistently demonstrates benefit in mortality, rebleeding rate, and functional status, and only one study provides comparison to medical management. No significant studies utilizing craniopuncture have been conducted in the USA.

Stereotactic Evacuation with Thrombolysis

The first major trial to evaluate the effect of stereotactic hematoma aspiration in conjunction with direct thrombolysis was the SICHPA trial (Stereotactic Treatment of Intracerebral Hematoma by Means of a Plasminogen Activator) in 2003 [10]. This trial compared stereotactic hematoma evacuation with urokinase to the best medical management. A catheter was inserted stereotactically and serially infused with urokinase to drain the hematoma over 48 hours. Seventy-one patients were randomly assigned to the surgical or nonsurgical groups. While there was no significant difference in mortality between the surgical and nonsurgical groups (56% vs 59%, respectively), there was a significant decrease in hematoma volume in the surgical arm over 7 days [10].

In the MISTIE trials (Minimally Invasive Surgery with Thrombolysis in Intracerebral hemorrhage Evacuation), surgical stereotactic hematoma evacuation with recombinant tissue plasminogen activator (rtPA) was compared to medical management. For their surgical technique, a sheath was stereotactically passed through a burr hole into the middle of the hematoma, and manual aspiration is performed. A catheter is then left behind in place of the sheath. The drainage catheter remains and periodic injection of alteplase is performed. Clot burden is assessed with daily CT scans, and injections continue until up to nine injections have been performed or the ICH volume is less than 15cm^3 [1, 11].

MISTIE-I (2008) provided hope for MIS treatment, as there was a significant increase in clot resolution compared to medical management, although it was only a phase 1 trial [11]. MISTIE-II (2016) was a multicenter phase II randomized trial comparing stereotactic aspiration with thrombolysis to conservative medical management in 96 patients and primarily focused on safety outcomes. There was no significant difference in the primary outcomes of 30-day mortality, periprocedural mortality, symptomatic bleeding, and infection leading them to conclude that MIS with alteplase was a safe technique [11].

MISTIE-III (2019) was a multicenter, blinded endpoint randomized controlled trial conducted in 506 patients. This efficacy study showed a decrease in length of hospital stay and mortality after 1 year compared to medical management with no significant difference in mRS at 1 year. However, for those patients who achieved a reduction in hematoma volume less than 15 mL, there was a significant improvement in mRS at 1 year [12]. Other trials of stereotactic aspiration with thrombolysis rarely demonstrated any positive effects; this in tandem with the exploratory nature of the MISTIE trials suggests a continued need to evaluate other surgical modalities [1].

Endoport-Mediated Evacuation

For this technique, a small craniotomy and dural opening is performed. An endoport along with its obturator is inserted into the hematoma. The obturator is removed, and hematoma evacuation is then performed with a microsurgical approach or with a handpiece allowing for suction, irrigation, and coagulation of vessels for hemostasis. The endoport is removed at the conclusion of the case [1]. Many different clinical studies have been conducted to evaluate an endoport-mediated system for ICH evacuation with the potential benefits including less tissue damage, better access and visualization for deep ICH, and potentially faster evacuation times.

The Early Minimally-Invasive Removal of ICH (ENRICH) trial is a recently resulted trial evaluating endoport-mediated hematoma evacuation using the BrainPath and Myriad devices. Prior to ENRICH, there have been small retrospective studies of endoport-mediated evacuation, although the results of those studies are inconclusive given that they either did not compare their experimental group to a control, had relatively small series of patients [13–15], or demonstrated poor functional outcomes [16]. They did, however, demonstrate potential positive outcomes in terms of the reduction of hematoma volume using an endoport-mediated evacuation system [13–15].The ENRICH trial published results with Bayesian analysis showing a posterior probability of superiority of surgery over medical management of 0.981. This was based off of a utility-weighted modified Rankin scale (uw-mRS) of 0.458 for the surgery group and 0.374 for the control group. While ICH in the general population is predominantly located within the basal ganglia, the trial ratio was roughly 70/30 lobar to basal ganglia because of an adaptive trial design. Anterior basal ganglia hemorrhages were dropped from enrollment when an interim analysis showed that the trial was unlikely to prove an effect with hemorrhages of that location. Therefore, the positivity of the trail overall was carried by the lobar hemorrhages. Nevertheless, ENRICH represents the first large, randomized controlled trial showing positive results for surgical intervention in ICH [17].

Endoscope-Assisted Evacuation

In this technique, an endoscope is combined with an aspiration cannula through an access sheath to remove the ICH via a small craniectomy. The endoscope provides visualization, while the cannula allows for aspiration and irrigation of the hematoma. This technique also allows for the coagulation of vessels for hemostasis. A drainage catheter can be left in the cavity as needed [1].

Auer et al. conducted a randomized controlled study in 100 patients with spontaneous supratentorial ICH and compared endoscopic hematoma evacuation with medical management. Patients in the surgical arm demonstrated significantly lower mortality rates at 6 months (30% vs 70%) and significant neurological functional improvement; however, it should be noted that the surgical outcome of those patients suffering a thalamic ICH was no different from those managed conservatively [18]. Other retrospective endoscopic studies generally demonstrated some benefit to this technique over medical management (e.g., lower rebleeding rate, decreased mortality, lower mRS score, improved functional outcomes, and/or greater evacuation percentages) [18–23]. In addition, two recent meta-analyses of this technique have been conducted which also demonstrate benefit [24, 25].

The Intraoperative Stereotactic Computed Tomography-Guided Endoscopic Surgery (ICES) for Brain Hemorrhage was a multicenter, randomized controlled trial which compared endoscopic hematoma evacuation to medical management. In this trial, 20 enrolled subjects were randomized into a surgical ($n = 14$) and control ($n = 6$) group. In addition, 36 subjects from the medical arm of the MISTIE trials were prospectively added to the control group for analysis. Their data suggests that endoscopic hematoma evacuation may improve functional outcomes, as the percentage of subjects with a mRS < 4 at 1 year was 42.9% and 23.7% for the surgical and control groups, respectively. However, with a high p-value ($p = 0.19$), these results are inconclusive. A large-scale clinical trial will need to be conducted to demonstrate true efficacy of endoscopic hematoma evacuation, as many of the aforementioned studies were conducted retrospectively or have small sample sizes.

Adjunctive Aspiration Devices

An adjunctive aspiration device functions similarly to an endoscope-assisted technique but with enhanced control over aspiration strength, potentially decreasing inadvertent damage to the adjacent normal brain parenchyma while enabling more thorough clot removal [1, 26]. These systems use an endoscope working channel for irrigation and another channel for a tool that combines aspiration and agitation of the clot. The Apollo system (Penumbra Inc., Alameda, California) is a low-profile system that consists of an aspiration wand which vibrates and softens the clot preventing the cannula from obstructing. The Artemis system (Penumbra Inc., Alameda, California) is the second-generation system. The set up for such a procedure requires neuronavigation, the endoscope and monitor, basic surgical instruments and the Artemis device with suction. Imaging is usually performed to check hematoma evacuation prior to closure, which generally requires angio equipment, a portable CT scanner or a burr hole ultrasound probe. Figure 2.1 shows an example of this procedure set up in the angiogram suite. In Fig. 2.2, the surgeon holds the endoscope and the aspiration device. The authors' preference is to have the assistance hold the endoscope sheath rather than staple it to the scalp, so that it can be manipulated as needed throughout the procedure. An example of the endoscope view during hematoma evacuation is shown in Fig. 2.3.

The Stereotactic ICH Underwater Blood Aspiration (SCUBA) method, using the Apollo system, was described by Kellner et al. The SCUBA technique occurs in two stages. In the first stage, the endoscope and adjunctive aspiration device are inserted, and high-power suction is applied at the depth of the hematoma. The endoscope and adjunctive aspiration device are then pulled back until it is at the proximal end of the hematoma. The suction is then decreased, and the irrigation is increased in order to expand the

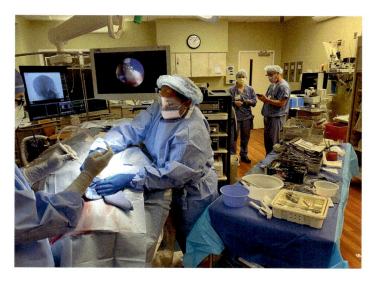

Fig. 2.1 Room set up for endoscopic assisted MIS ICH evacuation. This example is set up in the angiogram suite, demonstrating the endoscope tower, standard angiogram equipment and surgical back table. The stealth machine is also in-room, situated behind the camera in this instance

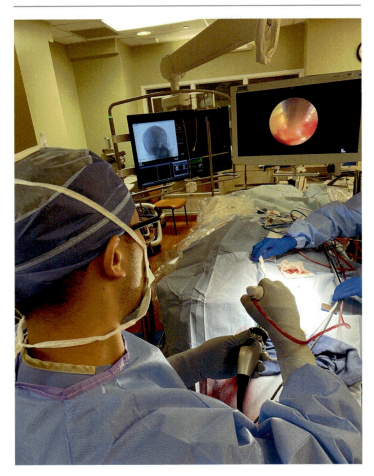

Fig. 2.2 View of the surgeon controlling both the aspiration device and the endoscope. In this situation, an assistant would control the depth of the sheath. The author's preference is for the surgeon to control both the endoscope and the sheath, with the resident or assistant controlling the aspiration device

cavity allowing for direct visualization and exploration of the cavity to allow for further clot evacuation as well as hemostasis. This second phase also helps to reduce trauma to cavity walls. The endoscope is then removed [1, 27].

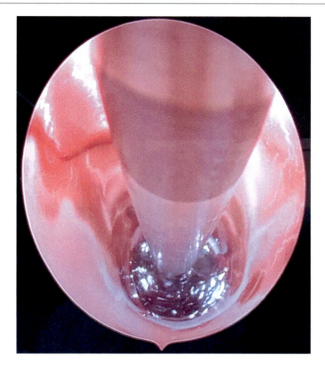

Fig. 2.3 Endoscope view during clot aspiration. In general, keeping the aspiration device advanced a clear distance out through the endoscope will help to keep the lens of the endoscope clean and maintain visualization. The authors also find that the 30 degree scope is not only manageable but may be easier in this regard.

Spiotta et al. reported on a multicenter initial experience utilizing the Apollo system in 29 patients demonstrating a significant reduction in hematoma size postoperatively [28]. Goyal et al. reported a case-control study of 19 patients who underwent MIS using the Apollo system of basal ganglia ICH. This interventional cohort was then matched to 54 conservatively managed patients. This series demonstrated a significantly lower in-hospital mortality in the MIS group (28% vs 56%) [29]. Figures 2.4a, b show pre-

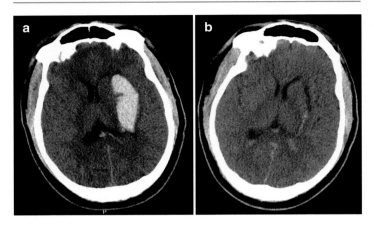

Fig. 2.4 (**a**) Head CT from a 48-year-old patient with a left external capsule hemorrhage. The patient required intubation for somnolence/airway protection and required drips to control blood pressure. (**b**) Postop head CT from the same patient after endoscopic-assisted MIS ICH evacuation. This was done through a burr hole on the left forehead. The patient was able to be extubated POD#1 and was transferred out of the ICU POD#3 once his blood pressure was controlled without IV drips. There were no issues with cerebral edema during his hospital stay

operative and postoperative CT scans for a patient with left side anterior basal ganglia ICH that was evacuated using an endoscope and adjunctive aspiration device via a burr hole placed on the left forehead.

The ongoing trials for adjunctive aspiration devices are the Minimally Invasive Endoscopic Surgery with Apollo in Patients with Brain Hemorrhage (INVEST) study which is based in the USA and the Dutch Intracerebral Hemorrhage Surgery Trial (DIST) based in the Netherlands. The results of these studies are not yet available. The Artemis in the Removal of Intracerebral Hemorrhage (MIND) study stopped enrollment early after the ENRICH trial results were released. This was done after enrollment of 236 patients, with interim analysis prespecified at an N of 200. The primary endpoint of the trial was mRS at 180 days and in this measure, the trial showed no difference between medical management and minimally invasive surgery (MIS) evacuation (OR 1.03; 96% CI, 0.62 to 1.72, P=0.452). However, the trial did show reduced perihematomal edema and reduced ventilator dependence at 30 days as well as reduced serious adverse events with MIS evacuation of ICH. It should be noted that MIND patients were split roughly 70/30 with most patients having basal ganglia hemorrhages, which is more reflective of the general population and is the inverse of the patients enrolled in ENRICH. At the time of this writing, the full results of the MIND trial are not yet published.

Surgiscope

The Aurora Surgiscope System is a relatively newer instrument. It is a single-use endoscope approved by the FDA in January of 2019. There are no published reports of techniques using this system yet. The Minimally Invasive Intracerebral Hemorrhage Evacuation (MIRROR) and Ultra-Early, Minimally Invasive Intracerebral Hemorrhage Evacuation Versus Standard Treatment (EVACUATE) trials have recently begun enrolling patients and should provide a better understanding around the efficacy of this technique [1].

Other Techniques

Other techniques to improve hematoma evacuation, such as transcatheter sonothrombolysis, have been reported but are not common in clinical practice [30].

Operative Setting and Intraoperative Imaging

As the field of neurointervention continues to expand, advancements in cone beam CT (CBCT) imaging have allowed for the evacuation of ICH in a minimally invasive manner with the assistance of real-time image guidance, thereby increasing the extent of the initial clot removal [26]. Many institutions utilizing adjunctive aspiration devices use them in hybrid or intraoperative angiography suites where CBCT allows for immediate feedback on the extent of hematoma evacuation.

Both the operating room and the angiography suite can be used as the setting for MIS ICH evacuation. Each has its own positive and negative considerations, but the key secondary decision is which type of imaging will be used to assess the clot evacuation mid-procedure. Given the subgroup analysis of MISTIE III showing that residual hematoma volume <15 cc may be associated with improved mRS at 1 year, it seems imperative that the clot evacuation be assessed mid-procedure, so that continued efforts can be made until that goal is reached. This is most commonly done in the angiography suite with CBCT but can also be done with a burr hole ultrasound (US) probe. In the operating room, the US probe is clearly still an option, but CT is only feasible if the institution possesses a portable CT technology, or the room is a hybrid suite.

Conclusions

MIS techniques offer several promising options for treating spontaneous intracerebral hemorrhage, although there is not yet a clinical study that suggests a definitive surgical advantage or an optimal surgical technique for treating this disease. There are, however, several ongoing clinical trials that are researching different MIS-ICH evacuation techniques that should help provide clarity around the efficacy of certain techniques and hopefully patient selection.

References

1. Musa MJ, Carpenter AB, Kellner C, Sigounas D, Godage I, Sengupta S, et al. Minimally invasive intracerebral hemorrhage evacuation: a review. Ann Biomed Eng. 2022;50:365–86.
2. Wu G, Li C, Wang L, Mao Y, Hong Z. Minimally invasive procedures for evacuation of intracerebral hemorrhage reduces perihematomal glutamate content, blood-brain barrier permeability and brain edema in rabbits. Neurocrit Care. 2011;14:118–26.

3. Mendelow AD, Gregson BA, Fernandes HM, Murray GD, Teasdale GM, Terence Hope D, et al. Early surgery versus initial conservative treatment in patients with spontaneous supratentorial intracerebral haematomas in the International Surgical Trial in Intracerebral Haemorrhage (STICH): a randomised trial. Lancet. 2005;365:387–97.
4. Mendelow AD, Gregson BA, Rowan EN, Murray GD, Gholkar A, Mitchell PM, et al. Early surgery versus initial conservative treatment in patients with spontaneous supratentorial lobar intracerebral haematomas (STICH II): a randomised trial. Lancet. 2013;382:397–408.
5. Wu G, Zhong W. Effect of minimally invasive surgery for cerebral hematoma evacuation in different stages on motor evoked potential and thrombin in dog model of intracranial hemorrhage. Neurol Res. 2010;32:127–33.
6. Scaggiante J, Zhang X, Mocco J, Kellner CP. Minimally invasive surgery for Intracerebral hemorrhage an updated meta-analysis of randomized controlled trials. Stroke. 2018;49:2612–20.
7. Sun H, Liu H, Li D, Liu L, Yang J, Wang W. An effective treatment for cerebral hemorrhage: minimally invasive craniopuncture combined with urokinase infusion therapy. Neurol Res. 2010;32:371–7.
8. Wang WZ, Jiang B, Liu HM, Li D, Lu CZ, Du Zhao Y, et al. Minimally invasive craniopuncture therapy vs. conservative treatment for spontaneous intracerebral hemorrhage: results from a randomized clinical trial in China. Int J Stroke. 2009;4:11–6.
9. Zhou H, Zhang Y, Liu L, Han X, Tao Y, Tang Y, et al. A prospective controlled study: minimally invasive stereotactic puncture therapy versus conventional craniotomy in the treatment of acute intracerebral hemorrhage. BMC Neurol. 2011; https://doi.org/10.1186/1471-2377-11-76.
10. Teernstra OPM, Evers SMAA, Lodder J, Leffers P, Franke CL, Blaauw G. Stereotactic treatment of intracerebral hematoma by means of a plasminogen activator: a multicenter randomized controlled trial (SICHPA). Stroke. 2003;34:968–74.
11. Morgan T, Zuccarello M, Narayan R, Keyl P, Lane K, Hanley D. Preliminary findings of the minimally-invasive surgery plus rtPA for intracerebral hemorrhage evacuation (MISTIE) clinical trial. Acta Neurochir Suppl (Wien). 2008;105:147.
12. Hanley DF, Thompson RE, Muschelli J, Rosenblum M, McBee N, Lane K, et al. Safety and efficacy of minimally invasive surgery plus alteplase in intracerebral haemorrhage evacuation (MISTIE): a randomised, controlled, open-label, phase 2 trial. Lancet Neurol. 2016;15:1228–37.
13. Przybylowski CJ, Ding D, Starke RM, Webster Crowley R, Liu KC. Endoport-assisted surgery for the management of spontaneous intracerebral hemorrhage. J Clin Neurosci. 2015;22:1727–32.
14. Bauer AM, Rasmussen PA, Bain MD. Initial single-center technical experience with the BrainPath system for acute intracerebral hemorrhage evacuation. Oper Neurosurg. 2017;13:69–76.
15. Labib M, Shah M, Kassam A, Young R, Zucker L, Maioriello A, et al. The safety and feasibility of image-guided brainpath-mediated Transsulcul Hematoma evacuation: a multicenter study, vol. 80. Neurosurgery; 2017. p. 515.

16. Griessenauer C, Medin C, Goren O, Schirmer CM. Image-guided, minimally invasive evacuation of Intracerebral Hematoma: a matched Cohort study comparing the endoscopic and tubular exoscopic systems. Cureus. 2018; https://doi.org/10.7759/cureus.3569.
    Pradilla G, Ratcliff JJ, Hall AJ, Saville BR, Allen JW, Paulon G, et al. ENRICH trial investigators; ENRICH Trial Investigators. Trial of Early Minimally Invasive Removal of Intracerebral Hemorrhage. N Engl J Med.   2024;390(14):1277–1289.   https://doi.org/10.1056/NEJMoa2308440. PMID: 38598795.

17. Auer LM, Deinsberger W, Niederkorn K, Gell G, Kleinert R, Schneider G, et al. Endoscopic surgery versus medical treatment for spontaneous intracerebral hematoma: a randomized study. J Neurosurg. 1989;70:530–5.

18. Nagasaka T, Tsugeno M, Ikeda H, Okamoto T, Inao S, Wakabayashi T. Early recovery and better evacuation rate in neuroendoscopic surgery for spontaneous intracerebral hemorrhage using a multifunctional cannula: preliminary study in comparison with craniotomy. J Stroke Cerebrovasc Dis. 2011;20:208–13.

19. Xu X, Chen X, Li F, Zheng X, Wang Q, Sun G, et al. Effectiveness of endoscopic surgery for supratentorial hypertensive intracerebral hemorrhage: a comparison with craniotomy. J Neurosurg. 2018;128:553–9.

20. Wang WH, Hung YC, Hsu SPC, Lin CF, Chen HH, Shih YH, et al. Endoscopic hematoma evacuation in patients with spontaneous supratentorial intracerebral hemorrhage. J Chin Med Assoc. 2015;78:101–7.

21. Cai Q, Zhang H, Zhao D, Yang Z, Hu K, Wang L, et al. Analysis of three surgical treatments for spontaneous supratentorial intracerebral hemorrhage. Medicine. 2017;96:1–9.

22. Vespa P, Hanley D, Betz J, Hoffer A, Engh J, Carter R, et al. ICES (Intraoperative Stereotactic Computed Tomography-Guided Endoscopic Surgery) for brain hemorrhage: a multicenter randomized controlled trial. Stroke. 2016;47:2749–55.

23. Nam T, Kim Y. A meta-analysis for evaluating efficacy of neuroendoscopic surgery versus craniotomy for supratentorial hypertensive intracerebral hemorrhage. J Cerebrovasc Endovasc Neurosurg. 2019;21:11.

24. Ye Z, Ai X, Hu X, Fang F, You C. Comparison of neuroendoscopic surgery and craniotomy for supratentorial hypertensive intracerebral hemorrhage. Medicine. 2017; https://doi.org/10.1097/MD.0000000000007876.

25. Fiorella D, Arthur A, Schafer S. Minimally invasive cone beam CT-guided evacuation of parenchymal and ventricular hemorrhage using the Apollo system: proof of concept in a cadaver model. J NeuroIntervent Surg. 2015;7:569–73.

26. Kellner CP, Chartrain AG, Nistal DA, Scaggiante J, Hom D, Ghatan S, et al. The Stereotactic Intracerebral Hemorrhage Underwater Blood Aspiration (SCUBA) technique for minimally invasive endoscopic intracerebral hemorrhage evacuation. J NeuroIntervent Surg. 2018;10:771–6.

27. Spiotta AM, Fiorella D, Vargas J, Khalessi A, Hoit D, Arthur A, et al. Initial multicenter technical experience with the Apollo device for minimally invasive intracerebral hematoma evacuation. Neurosurgery. 2015;11(Suppl 2):243–51. discussion 251

28. Goyal N, Tsivgoulis G, Malhotra K, Katsanos AH, Pandhi A, Alsherbini KA, et al. Minimally invasive endoscopic hematoma evacuation vs best medical management for spontaneous basal-ganglia intracerebral hemorrhage. J NeuroIntervent Surg. 2019;11:579–83.

29. Newell DW, Shah MM, Wilcox R, Hansmann DR, Melnychuk E, Muschelli J, et al. Minimally invasive evacuation of spontaneous intracerebral hemorrhage using sonothrombolysis: clinical article. J Neurosurg. 2011;115:592–601.

Middle Meningeal Artery Embolization for Chronic Subdural Hematoma

Alina Mohanty and Peter Kan

Chronic subdural hematomas (cSDHs) are one of the most encountered neurosurgical conditions; overall incidence is cited between 1.7 and 20.6 per 100,000 persons and as high as 79.4 per 100,000 hospital admissions in the Veteran Affairs population [1, 2]. As the population ages and as antiplatelet and anticoagulation medications become more prevalent, chronic subdural hematoma evacuation is expected to become the most common cranial neurosurgical operation in the adult population by 2030 [2]. CSDHs are originally thought to be the result of shearing of bridging veins after a minor trauma but are now believed to be a result of injury to the inner dural border cells, leading to an inflammatory response which contributes to the formation of neo-membranes and a recurring cycle of angiogenesis, inflammation, and hemolysis [3, 4]. Pathological neoangiogenesis and the creation of frail microvessels (with supply believed to originate from the middle meningeal artery, MMA) that rupture subsequently contribute to the cSDH overtime [5, 6]. Not all cSDHs require treatment—many are

A. Mohanty
Baylor College of Medicine Department of Neurosurgery,
Houston, TX, USA

P. Kan (✉)
Neurosurgery, The University of Texas Medical Branch at Galveston,
Galveston, TX, USA
e-mail: ptkan@utmb.edu

E. Veznedaroglu (ed.), *Advanced Technologies in Vascular
Neurosurgery*, https://doi.org/10.1007/978-3-031-67492-1_3

asymptomatic; medical management can include corticosteroids, antifibrinolytics, statins, and angiotensin-converting enzyme inhibitors; studies have yielded mixed results, and none of the above are standard of care at this time [7, 8]. However, if symptomatic or radiographically prominent (>10 mm in greatest thickness or with >5 mm of midline shift), surgical treatment is usually necessitated. The mass effect of the chronic subdural hematoma can result in altered mental status, seizures, weakness or sensory changes, and nausea/vomiting that lead to initial presentation. Despite initial surgical evacuation, recurrence rates of cSDHs have been noted to be anywhere from 10.9% to 26.3% [9].

Though treated traditionally by burr-hole evacuation, twist drill craniostomy with drainage, or craniotomy, middle meningeal artery embolization (MMAE) has developed in the last decade as a treatment and prevention of recurrent cSDHs. Studies such as those by Tanaka et al. [10] were published that angiographically demonstrated the middle meningeal artery (MMA) feeding into the outer membranes of cSDHs [10, 11]. First described by Mandai et al. [11] in 2000, middle meningeal artery embolization (MMAE) was attempted in a coagulopathic patient with low platelets and liver cirrhosis who continued to have recurrent cSDHs despite multiple surgical interventions. After embolization of the MMA and small volume evacuations of the hematoma with an Ommaya reservoir placed previously, serial CT scans demonstrated resolution of the cSDH after 7 months with no recurrence. Other initial case series published between 2002 and 2015 showed no recurrence of cSDHs [12–16]. Since those initial studies, several multicenter case series have demonstrated good results of MMA embolization; Kan et al. [17] published a case series in 2021 of 138 patients, of which 71% of patients had >50% radiographic improvement, 32% improved clinically, and 7% of patients required further treatment [17]. Other large case series by Rajah et al. [18], Link et al. [19], Ban et al. [20], Shotar et al. [21] and Joyce et al. [22] all demonstrated good outcomes—either with high percentage of stability/improvement in cSDH or small percentage of recurrences [18–22]. In summary, all these studies showed technical feasibility in majority (>90%) of cases and that the recurrence rate after MMAE (standalone or adjunct) is low (5–10%).

The middle meningeal artery is the dominant supply of the cranial dura. It can also supply portions of the falx cerebri, middle cranial fossa, anterior cranial fossa, and cavernous sinus. Though it most often arises from the external carotid artery as a branch of the maxillary artery, it can also arise from the internal carotid artery (ICA) or even the basilar artery [23]. The middle meningeal artery gives off two branches, the petrosal and cavernous branches, which supply the petrosal dura/tympanic cavity and the cavernous sinus, respectively, prior to dividing into the anterior and posterior divisions. The anterior division comprises falcine arteries and contralateral branches; the posterior division has two principal branches—the petrosquamosal branch and parieto-occipital branch. Because the MMA traverses through a large dural distribution, the MMA has possible anastomoses with arteries that originate from the ICA, ECA, and the vertebrobasilar system. These include anastomoses with the caroticotympanic artery, branches of the ascending pharyngeal artery, branches of the occipital artery, the inferolateral trunk, and branches of the ophthalmic artery: the recurrent meningeal artery of the ophthalmic artery and dural branches of the ophthalmic artery such as the anterior and posterior ethmoidal arteries, as well as the contralateral MMA [23, 24].

Due to the minimally invasive nature of the procedure, this procedure can be performed without general anesthesia and with minimal sedation and local anesthetic. Arterial access should be obtained through either the common femoral artery or radial artery, per the patient's anatomy and provider's experience. Next, a guide catheter should be inserted into the distal common carotid or proximal external carotid. The authors recommend visualizing the origin of the MMA, existing collaterals, and any possible dangerous anastomoses that might be present with the MMA. It should also be confirmed that the ophthalmic artery originates from the internal carotid artery (ICA) by observing retinal blush from an ICA injection. At this time, a microcatheter should be used to advance into the MMA for super-selective angiography, and any collaterals from the MMA such as meningolacrimal or meningo-ophthalmic branches should be identified so that embolization can occur distal to the location of these collaterals. Any anastomosis to the ophthalmic artery creates a risk for inadvertent embolization of that artery leading to blindness. Anastomoses with the cavernous branch of the MMA and the inferolateral trunk can supply Meckel's cave, with embolization of this collateral risking cranial nerve 5 injury [25], leading to facial numbness. Embolization of anastomoses to the petrosal branch that supplies the vasa vasorum of cranial nerve VII can cause facial paralysis. For this reason, many neurointerventionists will only embolize distal to the foramen spinosum. Ideally, the frontal and parietal branches of the MMA are embolized separately, distal to the bifurcation. MMA embolization in the MMA contralateral to the chronic subdural can also be performed, especially if there are noted collaterals from the contralateral MMA to MMA ipsilateral to the site of the chronic subdural. Embolic options include particles, Onyx, N-butyl cyanoacrylate (NBCA), other liquid embolics (e.g., SQUID), and coils. While liquid embolics are the most penetrating of distal branches, they are also the most likely to invertedly embolize collaterals. Particles, especially those larger in size 250–500 microns, are less likely to penetrate such collaterals. Embolization should persist until contrast opacification is obtained in the frontal and parietal branches of the MMA, and there is no further anterograde flow. Carotid angiography can be repeated at this stage to revisualize all intracranial vasculature. Repeat CT imaging is usually obtained 1–3 months after embolization, since MMA embolization has been shown to require at least 4–6 weeks for resolution of cSDH [17, 20].

Because cSDHs can take up to a few months to resolve with MMA embolization, if acute intervention is needed, evacuation of the cSDH must be done operatively prior to MMA embolization. Benefits of the MMA embolization include the minimally invasive nature of the procedure, little or even no general or systemic anesthesia, and the ability to perform embolization in patients that are otherwise not good surgical candidates—be that due to significant comorbidities or coagulopathies that might preclude them from evacuation such as craniectomy. MMA embolization also provides a potential treatment for cSDHs that have been refractory to medical as well as repeated surgical treatment. MMA embolization is not possible if there is poor vascular access or any contraindications to contrast such as pregnancy, contrast allergy, or significant renal injury or disease. Significant coagulopathy might also hinder treatment via embolization. Risks associated with this procedure include those associated with diagnostic cerebral angiogram (i.e., groin/wrist hematoma, arterial injury, stroke, transient ischemic attack) as well as the complications associated with the embolization, most importantly unintentional embolization of other intracranial arteries and injury to the cranial nerves leading to blindness and facial paralysis, as discussed above.

We present the case of a 65-year-old male with cirrhosis secondary to hepatitis C and known bilateral subdural hygromas who presented with headaches after a fall a few days prior. His platelet count was 93, but his prothrombin time and partial thromboplastin time were within normal limits. He was neurologically intact on exam. CT imaging obtained demonstrated bilateral subdural isodense fluid collections approximately 16 mm on the left and 10 mm on the right with an associated 3.5 mm midline shift (Fig. 3.1a). He underwent bilateral MMA embolization; angiograms visualize right and left external carotid arteries before (Figs. 3.2a and 3.3a) and during (Figs. 3.2b, c and 3.3b, c) embolization with selective catheterization of frontal and parietal MMA branches. CT obtained 3 months after embolization (Fig. 3.1b) showed decrease in subdural hematoma size, and CT obtained 6 months after embolization (Fig. 3.1c) showed complete resolution of bilateral subdural hematomas.

With several case series demonstrating improvement of cSDH after embolization and little to no recurrences, several trials are

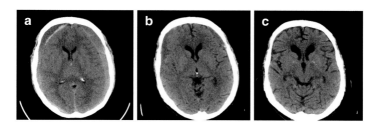

Fig. 3.1 (**a**) Prior to treatment, (**b**) 3 months after bilateral MMA embolization, and (**c**) 6 months after MMA embolization

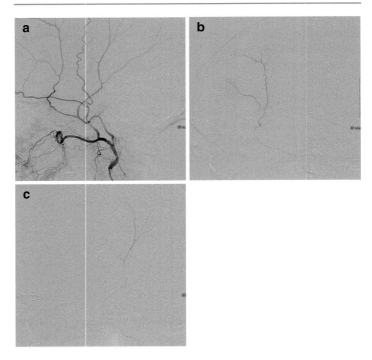

Fig. 3.2 (**a**) Right ECA prior to embolization and (**b**) selective catheterization of frontal and (**c**) parietal branch during MMA embolization. Abbreviations: ECA external carotid artery, MMA middle meningeal artery

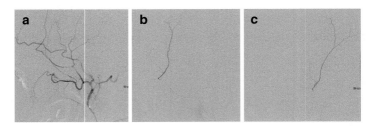

Fig. 3.3 (**a**) Left ECA prior to embolization and (**b**) selective catheterization of frontal and (**c**) parietal branch during MMA embolization. Abbreviations: ECA external carotid artery, MMA middle meningeal artery

ongoing to compare MMA embolization to conventional management. A meta-analysis published in 2023 by Sattari et al. [26] of nine studies and 1523 patients that compared MMA embolization to conventional management found that the relative risk of treatment failure in MMA embolization was significantly lower compared with conventional management (5.6% vs 22.2%, RR = 0.34 [0.14–0.82], $P = .02$, $I^2 = 64\%$, $P = .005$). Additionally, they found that the relative risk of surgical rescue was significantly lower after MMA embolization vs conventional management (4.1% vs 16.1%, RR = 0.33 [0.14–0.77], $P = .01$, $I^2 = 52\%$, $P = .030$) without any significant differences in relative risk of complications (8% vs 11.6%, RR = 0.93 [0.63–1.37], $P = .72$, $I^2 = 0$, $P = .58$). Another meta-analysis of 1416 patients—one group of 718 who underwent MMA embolization and another group of 698 who had conventional management—published by Ironside et al. [27] in 2021 similarly showed significantly decreased relative risks of cSDH recurrence and surgical rescue in the MMA embolization group without a significant difference in complications when compared to the conventional management group. There are now multiple ongoing randomized clinical trials in the United States that are comparing conventional management (whether that is both surgical and nonsurgical management or just conventional surgical management) to MMA embolization (most adjunctive with conventional management). Three of these trials are studying conventional management (both surgical and nonsurgical) vs conventional management in conjunction with MMA embolization with liquid embolics: Middle Meningeal Artery Embolization for the Treatment of Subdural Hematomas With TRUFILL® n-BCA (MEMBRANE) [28] with NBCA, SQUID Trial for the Embolization of the Middle Meningeal Artery for Treatment of Chronic Subdural Hematoma (STEM) [29] with SQUID, and Embolization of the Middle Meningeal Artery With ONYX™ Liquid Embolic System for Subacute and Chronic Subdural Hematoma (EMBOLISE) [30] with Onyx. The outcomes for all three trials measure hematoma recurrence but vary in their additional outcome measures. The upcoming Chronic Subdural Hematoma Treatment with Embolization vs Surgery Study

(CHESS) trial will study conventional surgical management vs primary MMA embolization without any adjunctive treatment, using PVA or Embospheres for embolization. Through these clinical trials, we can begin to understand the extent of the effectiveness of MMA embolization and greater understand for which patients MMA embolization will be the most suitable. With these studies and additional studies, we can also further study the effectiveness and safety of the different embolics, techniques, and treatment criteria. If these randomized clinical trials continue to show benefit of MMA embolization compared to conventional treatment, we can expect to see MMA embolization become standard of care in the coming years for treatment of cSDHs.

References

1. Feghali J, Yang W, Huang J. Updates in chronic subdural hematoma: epidemiology, etiology, pathogenesis, treatment, and outcome. World Neurosurg.   2020;141:339–45.   https://doi.org/10.1016/j. wneu.2020.06.140. Epub 2020 Jun 25. PMID: 32593768.
2. Balser D, Farooq S, Mehmood T, Reyes M, Samadani U. Actual and projected incidence rates for chronic subdural hematomas in United States Veterans Administration and civilian populations. J Neurosurg. 2015;123:1209–15.
3. Sahyouni R, Goshtasbi K, Mahmoodi A, Tran DK, Chen JW. Chronic subdural hematoma: a historical and clinical perspective. World Neurosurg. 2017;108:948–53.
4. Katano H, Kamiya K, Mase M, Tanikawa M, Yamada K. Tissue plasminogen activator in chronic subdural hematomas as a predictor of recurrence. J Neurosurg. 2006;104:79–84.
5. Weigel R, Hohenstein A, Schilling L. Vascular endothelial growth factor concentration in chronic subdural hematoma fluid is related to computed tomography appearance and exudation rate. J Neurotrauma. 2014;31:670–3.
6. Kalamatianos T, Stavrinou LC, Koutsarnakis C, Psachoulia C, Sakas DE, Stranjalis G. PlGF and sVEGFR-1 in chronic subdural hematoma: implications for hematoma development. J Neurosurg. 2013;118:353–7.
7. Roh D, Reznik M, Claassen J. Chronic subdural medical management. Neurosurg Clin N Am. 2017;28:211–7.
8. Hutchinson PJ, Edlmann E, Bulters D, Zolnourian A, Holton P, Suttner N, Agyemang K, Thomson S, Anderson IA, Al-Tamimi YZ, Henderson D, Whitfield PC, Gherle M, Brennan PM, Allison A, Thelin EP, Tarantino S, Pantaleo B, Caldwell K, Davis-Wilkie C, Mee H, Warburton EA, Barton

G, Chari A, Marcus HJ, King AT, Belli A, Myint PK, Wilkinson I, Santarius T, Turner C, Bond S, Kolias AG. British Neurosurgical Trainee Research Collaborative; Dex-CSDH Trial Collaborators. Trial of Dexamethasone for chronic subdural hematoma. N Engl J Med. 2020;383(27):2616–27. https://doi.org/10.1056/NEJMoa2020473. Epub 2020 Dec 16. PMID: 33326713.

9. Zhu F, Wang H, Li W, Han S, Yuan J, Zhang C, Li Z, Fan G, Liu X, Nie M, Bie L. Factors correlated with the postoperative recurrence of chronic subdural hematoma: an umbrella study of systematic reviews and meta-analyses. EClinicalMedicine. 2021;43:101234. https://doi.org/10.1016/j.eclinm.2021.101234. PMID: 34988412; PMCID: PMC8703229

10. Tanaka T, Fujimoto S, Saito K, et al. Histological study of operated cases of chronic subdural hematoma in adults: relationship between dura mater and outer membrane. No Shinkei Geka. 1997;25:701–705. (Jpn)

11. Mandai S, Sakurai M, Matsumoto Y. Middle meningeal artery embolization for refractory chronic subdural hematoma. Case report. J Neurosurg. 2000;93(4):686–8. https://doi.org/10.3171/jns.2000.93.4.0686. PMID: 11014549.

12. Ishihara H, Ishihara S, Kohyama S, Yamane F, Ogawa M, Sato A, Matsutani M. Experience in endovascular treatment of recurrent chronic subdural hematoma. Interv Neuroradiol. 2007;13(Suppl 1):141–4.

13. Tempaku A, Yamauchi S, Ikeda H, Tsubota N, Furukawa H, Maeda D, Kondo K, Nishio A. Usefulness of interventional embolization of the middle meningeal artery for recurrent chronic subdural hematoma: five cases and a review of the literature. Interv Neuroradiol. 2015;21:366–71.

14. Mino M, Nishimura S, Hori E, Kohama M, Yonezawa S, Midorikawa H, Kaimori M, Tanaka T, Nishijima M. Efficacy of middle meningeal artery embolization in the treatment of refractory chronic subdural hematoma. Surg Neurol Int. 2010;1:78.

15. Takahashi K, Muraoka K, Sugiura T, Maeda Y, Mandai S, Gohda Y, Kawauchi M, Matsumoto Y. Middle meningeal artery embolization for refractory chronic subdural hematoma: 3 case reports. No Shinkei Geka. 2002;30:535–9.

16. Hashimoto T, Ohashi T, Watanabe D, et al. Usefulness of embolization of the middle meningeal artery for refractory chronic subdural hematomas. Surg Neurol Int. 2013;4:104.

17. Kan P, Maragkos GA, Srivatsan A, Srinivasan V, Johnson J, Burkhardt JK, Robinson TM, Salem MM, Chen S, Riina HA, Tanweer O, Levy EI, Spiotta AM, Kasab SA, Lena J, Gross BA, Cherian J, Cawley CM, Howard BM, Khalessi AA, Pandey AS, Ringer AJ, Hanel R, Ortiz RA, Langer D, Kelly CM, Jankowitz BT, Ogilvy CS, Moore JM, Levitt MR, Binning M, Grandhi R, Siddiq F, Thomas AJ. Middle meningeal artery embolization for chronic subdural hematoma: a multi-center experience of 154 consecutive embolizations. Neurosurgery. 2021;88(2):268–77. https://doi.org/10.1093/neuros/nyaa379. PMID: 33026434.

18. Rajah GB, Waqas M, Dossani RH, et al. Transradial middle meningeal artery embolization for chronic subdural hematoma using Onyx: case series. J Neurointerv Surg. 2020;12:1214–8.

19. Link TW, Boddu S, Paine SM, Kamel H, Knopman J. Middle meningeal artery embolization for chronic subdural hematoma: a series of 60 cases. Neurosurgery. 2019;85:801–7.

20. Ban SP, Hwang G, Byoun HS, Kim T, Lee SU, Bang JS, Han JH, Kim C-Y, Kwon O-K, Oh CW. Middle meningeal artery embolization for chronic subdural hematoma. Radiology. 2018;286:992–9.

21. Shotar E, Meyblum L, Premat K, et al. Middle meningeal artery embolization reduces the post-operative recurrence rate of at-risk chronic subdural hematoma. J Neurointerv Surg. 2020;12:1209–13.

22. Joyce E, Bounajem MT, Scoville J, et al. Middle meningeal artery embolization treatment of nonacute subdural hematomas in the elderly: a multiinstitutional experience of 151 cases. Neurosurg Focus. 2020;49:E5.

23. Bonasia S, Smajda S, Ciccio G, Robert T. Middle meningeal artery: anatomy and variations. AJNR Am J Neuroradiol. 2020;41(10):1777–85. https://doi.org/10.3174/ajnr.A6739. Epub 2020 Sep 3. PMID: 32883667; PMCID: PMC7661066.

24. Martínez JL, Domingo RA, Sattur M, Porto G, Rivas GA, Al Kasab S, Spiotta A. The middle meningeal artery: branches, dangerous anastomoses, and implications in neurosurgery and neuroendovascular surgery. Oper Neurosurg (Hagerstown). 2022;22(1):1–13. https://doi.org/10.1227/ONS.0000000000000010. PMID: 34982899.

25. Shapiro M, Walker M, Carroll KT, Levitt MR, Raz E, Nossek E, Delavari N, Mir O, Nelson PK. Neuroanatomy of cranial dural vessels: implications for subdural hematoma embolization. J Neurointerv Surg. 2021;13(5):471–7. https://doi.org/10.1136/neurintsurg-2020-016798. Epub 2021 Feb 25. PMID: 33632880.

26. Sattari SA, Yang W, Shahbandi A, Feghali J, Lee RP, Xu R, Jackson C, Gonzalez LF, Tamargo RJ, Huang J, Caplan JM. Middle meningeal artery embolization versus conventional management for patients with chronic subdural hematoma: a systematic review and meta-analysis. Neurosurgery. 2023;92(6):1142–54. https://doi.org/10.1227/neu.0000000000002365. Epub 2023 Mar 17. PMID: 36929762.

27. Ironside N, Nguyen C, Do Q, Ugiliweneza B, Chen CJ, Sieg EP, James RF, Ding D. Middle meningeal artery embolization for chronic subdural hematoma: a systematic review and meta-analysis. J Neurointerv Surg. 2021;13(10):951–7. https://doi.org/10.1136/neurintsurg-2021-017352. Epub 2021 Jun 30. PMID: 34193592.

28. https://clinicaltrials.gov/study/NCT04816591 - MEMBRANE trial.

29. https://clinicaltrials.gov/study/NCT04410146 - STEM trial.

30. https://classic.clinicaltrials.gov/ct2/show/record/NCT04402632 - EMBOLISE trial.

Role of Bypass in the Modern Era: Technological Advancements in Adjuncts for EC-IC Bypass

4

Sanjana Salwi, Visish Srinivasan, and Jan-Karl Burkhardt

Effect of Technological Advances on EC-IC Bypass

The evolution of extracranial-intracranial bypass surgery has depended on advances in technology to improve surgical techniques and perioperative care. In the 1960s, the first human intracranial bypass procedures were facilitated by the introduction of the operative microscope. In 1961, Pool and Potts performed one of the first STA-ACA (superior temporal artery-anterior cerebral artery) bypasses using a plastic tube [1]. In close follow-up, in 1963, Woringer and Kunlin performed the first extracranial-intracranial (EC-IC) bypass using a saphenous vein graft [2]. Though the first procedure was complicated by graft occlusion and the second by patient mortality, this opened the stage for further refinement of microsurgical techniques [3].

Advances in neurosurgical tools including bipolar cautery, vascular clips and appliers, and improved control of operative micro-

S. Salwi (✉) · V. Srinivasan · J.-K. Burkhardt
University of Pennsylvania, Department of Neurosurgery, Philadelphia, PA, USA
e-mail: Sanjana.Salwi@Pennmedicine.upenn.edu

© The Author(s), under exclusive license to Springer Nature Switzerland AG 2025
E. Veznedaroglu (ed.), *Advanced Technologies in Vascular Neurosurgery*, https://doi.org/10.1007/978-3-031-67492-1_4

scope allowed for further development of bypass techniques. In 1972, Yasargil performed the first superior temporal artery-middle cerebral artery (STA-MCA) bypass for a 4-year-old boy with Moyamoya disease with excellent clinical improvement in his symptoms [4]. Later in the 1970s, improvement in operative adjuncts like hypothermia, intraoperative monitoring, and better anesthetic techniques allowed for an expansion in pathology treated by bypass [5].

In the modern era, the main indications for EC-IC bypass are for (1) cerebral blood flow augmentation in patients with chronic intracranial arterial stenosis or Moyamoya disease or for (2) cerebral blood flow replacement for treatment of complex aneurysms or for tumor surgery requiring vessel sacrifice [6]. Important technological adjuncts in the last few decades include intraoperative micro-Doppler ultrasonography and surgical microscope-based indocyanine green video angiography (ICG). Both allow for intraoperative confirmation of graft patency in addition or instead of intraoperative catheter angiogram.

As technology continues to improve, new adjuncts in the modern era further facilitate operative technique and allow for improved postoperative monitoring of complications. These advances will be the focus of this chapter.

Ushering in a New Era of Bypass with Technological Adjuncts

Augmented Reality

Given the complex anatomy, availability of multiple advanced imaging modalities, and delicate surgical techniques, neurosurgery is a field that readily lends itself to integration with augmented reality (AR). Present conventional neuro-navigation modalities display two-dimensional (2D) information requiring the surgeon to cognitively reformat imaging information while operating. Furthermore, since the images are often displayed on multiple screens separate from the operative field, the surgeon must continuously look away from the operative field to confirm navigation [7]. AR technology allows for direct overlay of three-dimensional (3D) imaging information within the operative field. This reduces the risk that the surgeon will need to look away from the operative field during a critical portion. Additionally, this technology simplifies the mental task of converting multiple 2D images into a 3D reconstruction and allows for seamless application of this new spatial model to real-time anatomy.

AR technology can be particularly useful for bypass procedures given the technical excellence with multiple microsurgical techniques needed to ensure durability of the graft. Highlighting important anatomical structure can reduce cognitive load on the surgeon and facilitate careful dissection. For example, key anatomical structures including the STA, preselected middle cerebral artery branch 4 (M4), middle meningeal artery (MMA), and primary motor cortex (PMC) can be manually or automatically segmented on various modalities including magnetic resonance imaging (MRI), computed tomography angiography (CTA), and digital subtraction angiography (DSA). Then, this multi-modality segmentation can be reconstructed into a 3D image and then overlaid directly onto the operative field allowing for anatomic mapping. Overlaying the tortuous course of the STA facilitates careful dissection and identification of branching vessels. AR can also assist with craniotomy planning including techniques to preserve the middle meningeal artery (MMA) and allow for duro-encephalo-synangiosis [8]. These overlays can be directly visualized under an operative microscope to allow surgeons to use this technology with minimal disruption to standard operative technique.

Role of Exoscope for Bypass Surgery

There are a few reports on using an exoscope instead of a microscope to improve surgical visibility and provide efficient ergonomics for the surgeon to minimize complications and maximize successful revascularization [9–11]. Despite the operative microscope's utilization improvements such as ICG and visualization improvements, there remains a need for continued improvement in operative visualization and surgical ergonomics for this challenging procedure [12]. Especially the 4K high-definition (4K-HD) three-dimensional (3D) exoscope (EX) seems a novel promising approach. In a retrospective study, feasibility was confirmed using this technique, and the lightweight design of the EX allowed for easy instrument maneuverability as well as uncomplicated surgical setup in the operating room as described by the authors [12]. Also, the assistance of the co-surgeon was more efficient compared to that of the operating microscope. The large monitor allowed for an immersive, collaborative, and valuable educational surgical experience.

Role of Sonolucent Cranioplasty

Careful postoperative monitoring of graft complications is essential after EC-IC bypass to identify occlusion, low flow states, and hyper-perfusion syndrome. Early graft occlusion (1 week) is a serious postoperative complication that has been reported to occur in as high as 5% of cases [13]. Imaging findings can precede clinical symptoms so early identification can allow for expedited intervention with intra-arterial vasodilator, balloon angioplasty, or open surgical re-exploration to establish graft patency.

Ultrasound monitoring offers numerous advantages over conventional CT angiography including avoidance of radiation exposure and speed. A significant innovation in this sphere is a sonolucent cranioplasty that allows for real-time ultrasound monitoring at bedside.

Operative Procedure and Postoperative Monitoring

Two types of poly-methyl-methylacrylate (PMMA) clear implants can be used—a custom-made one based on preoperative imaging and a standard curved plate [14]. Both can be easily modified intraoperatively. After the bypass procedure, patency of the vessel is confirmed using micro-Doppler probe and ICG angiography. A template for size and shape is created based on the removed bone flap. Then, using that template, the shape of the sonolucent cranioplasty is cut from the PMMA clear implant. This can then be fixed with a standard cranial plating system (Figs. 4.1 and 4.2d–e). At our institution, we make intraoperative modifications to a pre-made curved PMMA disc and then fix the implant with a combination of titanium dog bones and screws following dural closure with a dural substitute [3, 15, 16]. For all bypasses with sonolucent cranioplasty, the likely graft location can be marked immediately postoperatively using knowledge of graft location and other landmarks seen on intraoperative angiography.

Postoperative Monitoring

Doppler ultrasonography with the linear transducer is used to evaluate for patency of the vessel in the short-axis view, and general shape of graft can be elucidated with long-axis view (Fig. 4.1). Ultrasound offers a wealth of information past simple visualization of graft patency. Measurement at various depths allows for

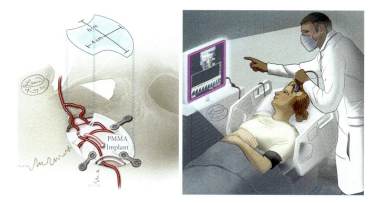

Fig. 4.1 Left: Graphic showing placement of PMMA implant with three points of fixation with titanium two-hole dog bone plate. Burr hole at inferior edge of skull defect allows for passage of bypass vessels. Right: Bedside visualization of vessels with transcranioplasty ultrasonography

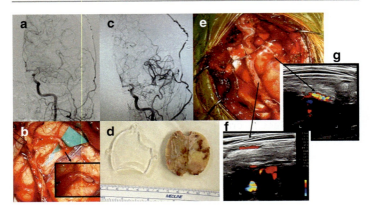

Fig. 4.2 Representative case for a patient with symptomatic Moyamoya disease who underwent a combined direct/indirect STA-MCA bypass. (**a**) Preoperative angiogram demonstrating L M1 occlusion and Moyamoya vessels. (**b**) Intraoperative photograph demonstrating bypass. (**c**) Intraoperative angiogram demonstrating patency of direct and indirect bypass. (**d**) PMMA implant was modeled from removed bone flap. (**e**) Implant is fixed in place with opening for bypass vessels. Transcranioplasty color Doppler sonography demonstrating patency of indirect bypass (**f**) and direct bypass (**g**)

measurement of graft velocity. Given the ease of measurement, this velocity can be trended daily to monitor for a sharp increase—which can signal partial stenosis. Further measurements can be performed easily at bedside to impute flow rate based on volumetric analysis and velocity measurements. In graft occlusion or severe vasospasm, there can be a significant decrease in flow rate that can precede clinical symptoms. Furthermore, long-axis views can provide further information on shape of vessel and can show graft kinking or areas of significant graft angulation. Further measurements can be made with spectral analysis with color Doppler to trend velocity and pulsatility index. These measurements provide a multifactorial and longitudinal picture of graft health. These measurements can be trended daily to evaluate for partial stenosis, occlusion, and hyper-perfusion to guide further imaging evaluation and potential operative intervention [17].

Patient Outcomes

In present literature on patient outcomes, there are no direct complications attributable to the PMMA implant. A recent multicenter study demonstrates safety of this novel implant as well as utility for post-procedure monitoring [17].

Furthermore, there are significant cost savings attributable to using a sonolucent cranioplasty. This cost saving is compounded given the amount of imaging these patients typically receive in the follow-up period. Three ultrasound studies at regular intervals during the follow-up period cost $900 compared to the standard follow-up imaging involving digital subtraction angiography and CT which can cost $11,000 in the follow-up period [16].

Conclusion

Technological advances continue to improve the intraoperative and postoperative tools to facilitate successful surgical revascularization. Three such notable advances are augmented reality with operative microscope, usage of exoscope, and ultrasound monitoring of graft through a sonolucent cranioplasty. Augmented reality allows for direct anatomical mapping overlaid on the surgical field through a now familiar operative adjunct—the surgical microscope. The exoscope offers improved surgical visibility and ergonomics. Sonolucent cranioplasty implant allows for a wealth of measurements in the immediate postoperative period and for long-term follow-up. Ultrasound monitoring allows for safe, real-time, efficient monitoring without exposing patients to ionizing radiation. It can be used to guide operative intervention for postoperative complications and for long-term follow-up.

Disclosures

SS: None
VS: None
JKB: Consultant: Stryker, Microvention, Cerenovus, Balt, Medtronic, Q'Apel Medical, Longeviti Neuro Solutions, Siemens Healthineers.

References

1. Pool JL, Potts DG. Aneurysms and Arteriovenous Anomalies of the brain: diagnosis and treatment. New York: Hoeber Medical Division, Harper & Row; 1965.
2. Woringer E, Kunlin J. Anastomosis between the common Carotid and the intracranial Carotid or the Sylvian artery by a graft, using the Suspended Suture Technic. Neurochirurgie. 1963;9:181–8.
3. Hadley C, North R, Srinivasan V, Kan P, Burkhardt JK. Elective Sonolucent Cranioplasty for real-time ultrasound monitoring of flow and patency of an extra- to intracranial bypass. J Craniofac Surg. 2020;31(3):622–4.
4. Krayenbuhl HA. The Moyamoya syndrome and the neurosurgeon. Surg Neurol. 1975;4(4):353–60.
5. Hayden MG, Lee M, Guzman R, Steinberg GK. The evolution of cerebral revascularization surgery. Neurosurg Focus. 2009;26(5):E17.
6. Burkhardt JK, Lawton MT. Practice trends in intracranial bypass surgery in a 21-year experience. World Neurosurg. 2019;125:e717–e22.
7. Pandya A, Siadat MR, Auner G. Design, implementation and accuracy of a prototype for medical augmented reality. Comput Aided Surg. 2005;10(1):23–35.
8. Rychen J, Goldberg J, Raabe A, Bervini D. Augmented reality in superficial temporal artery to middle cerebral artery bypass surgery: technical note. Oper Neurosurg (Hagerstown). 2020;18(4):444–50.
9. Belykh E, George L, Zhao X, Carotenuto A, Moreira LB, Yagmurlu K, et al. Microvascular anastomosis under 3D exoscope or endoscope magnification: a proof-of-concept study. Surg Neurol Int. 2018;9:115.
10. Hafez A, Haeren RHL, Dillmann J, Laakso A, Niemela M, Lehecka M. Comparison of operating microscope and exoscope in a highly challenging experimental setting. World Neurosurg. 2021;147:e468–e75.
11. Patel NV, Ligas B, Gandhi S, Ellis J, Ortiz R, Costantino P, et al. Internal maxillary to middle cerebral artery bypass using an anterior Tibial artery graft, performed using a 3-dimensional exoscope: 2-dimensional operative video. Oper Neurosurg (Hagerstown). 2020;19(2):E187.
12. Nossek E, Schneider JR, Kwan K, Kulason KO, Du V, Chakraborty S, et al. Technical aspects and operative Nuances using a high-definition 3-dimensional exoscope for cerebral bypass surgery. Oper Neurosurg (Hagerstown). 2019;17(2):157–63.
13. Yoon S, Burkhardt JK, Lawton MT. Long-term patency in cerebral revascularization surgery: an analysis of a consecutive series of 430 bypasses. J Neurosurg. 2018;131(1):80–7.
14. Rossitto CP, Devarajan A, Zhang JY, Benowitz R, Price G, Ali M, et al. Transcranioplasty ultrasonography through a Sonolucent prosthesis: a review of feasibility, safety, and benefits. World Neurosurg. 2023;178:152.

15. Flores AR, Srinivasan VM, Gadot R, Kan P, Burkhardt JK. Dural substitutes differentially interfere with imaging quality of Sonolucent Transcranioplasty ultrasound assessment in Benchtop model. World Neurosurg. 2020;144:e389–e94.

16. Flores AR, Srinivasan VM, Seeley J, Huggins C, Kan P, Burkhardt JK. Safety, feasibility, and patient-rated outcome of Sonolucent Cranioplasty in Extracranial-intracranial bypass surgery to allow for transcranioplasty ultrasound assessment. World Neurosurg. 2020;144:e277–e84.

17. Salem MM, Ravindran K, Hoang AN, Doron O, Esparza R, Raper D, et al. Sonolucent Cranioplasty in Extracranial to intracranial bypass surgery: early multicenter experience of 44 cases. Oper Neurosurg (Hagerstown). 2023;25(1):20–7.

Embolic Protection Devices for Carotid Artery Stenting: Where Is the Evidence?

5

Mohanad Sulaiman
and Mandy J. Binning

Introduction

Stroke is one of the most common causes of death and disability among all ages. Carotid artery disease (CAD) remains a common clinical entity that can lead to stroke. Present treatment options for CAD include open surgical carotid endarterectomy (CEA) or endovascular carotid artery stenting (CAS) via either a transfemoral (TFCAS) or transcarotid approach (TCAR). CEA and CAS are equivalent in long-term prevention of stroke ipsilateral to the treated carotid artery [1]. However, despite two decades of evolution, CAS has failed to be adopted as a superior alternative to CEA due to increased periprocedural stroke rates. Patients at high risk for CEA may be candidates for CAS. The decision to treat high-risk carotid stenosis by CEA or CAS is controversial. However, the most widely accepted indications for CAS are patients with clinically significant cardiac risk or those with high-risk neck anatomic features, including very high carotid bifurcation, restenosis following a prior CEA, or prior neck radiation.

M. Sulaiman · M. J. Binning (✉)
Global Neurosciences Institute (GNI), Drexel University,
Pennington, NJ, USA
e-mail: msulaiman@gnineuro.org; mbinning@gnineuro.org

CAS is also recommended for acute carotid occlusion especially in the presence of symptomatic acute occlusion with a large ischemic penumbra. CEA remains the standard of care in the treatment of CAD due to its ability to achieve flow arrest that prevents distal embolization of plaque particles from plaque disruption. If periprocedural stroke events occur, they are typically ipsilateral to the treated artery. The median time of stroke onset is zero days after the procedure, which suggests that these events are directly related to plaque characteristics and disruption as well as the manipulation of endovascular catheters and wires through the unprotected aortic arch or stenotic carotid artery [1]. In order to mitigate this risk, embolic protection devices (EPDs) were developed. The evolution of endovascular technology has included the development of a wide array of proximal and distal EPDs. More recently, transcarotid artery revascularization (TCAR) has been an option for CAS. Embolic protection devices (EPDs) can theoretically reduce periprocedural strokes. Although data regarding their effectiveness are controversial, and there is a lack of randomized controlled trials (RCTs) supporting the superiority of protected to unprotected CAS, EPDs have become the standard of care in CAS.

Embolic Protection Devices

Angioplasty for carotid bifurcation was first reported by Mathias and his colleagues in 1980. However, the risk of an embolic complication was extremely high (8–10%). Rapid improvement in endovascular technology resulted in the development of EPDs with different mechanisms for stroke prevention. Distal filter EPDs (F-EPDs) are small baskets deployed in the ICA distal to the lesion to catch any debris that may be produced by manipulation during angioplasty and stent placement. Proximal EPDs (P-EPDs) use balloons or flow-reversal mechanisms to arrest or reverse flow to the ICA so that angioplasty and stenting can be performed with reduced risk of antegrade embolization. Aspiration is performed either continuously or before balloon deflation to capture any debris released by the procedure. The indications for proximal versus distal protection use have yet to be clearly defined. In theory, intraluminal thrombus, vulnerable plaque, and poor distal landing zone anatomy would require proximal protection. Furthermore, the revolution that has ensued in the endovascular arena has yet to widely adopt newer protection techniques, such as transcarotid artery revascularization (TCAR). This is a relatively new procedure that combines the minimally invasive advantages of CAS while also using complete carotid artery blood flow reversal as neuroprotection. To briefly describe the procedure, embolic protection is accomplished by proximal carotid artery clamp placement followed by reversal of carotid artery blood flow through an extracorporeal circuit from the carotid artery to the femoral vein. This facilitates proximal protection, avoids traversing the aortic arch, allows retrograde removal of atherosclerotic debris, and establishes protection before manipulation of the carotid bifurcation lesion. This procedure will be described in greater detail at the end of this chapter.

To date, there have not been any RCTs comparing CAS with and without EPDs or any RCTs comparing the use of filters versus proximal balloon occlusion so far. Most evidence comes from studies using historical controls in the unprotected arm. In 2003, Kastrup et al. performed one of the earliest literature reviews to evaluate the efficacy of cerebral protection devices in preventing thromboembolic complications during CAS [2]. They evaluated the results of 40 CAS studies without cerebral protection and 14 CAS studies with protection. The stroke and death rate within 30 days was 1.8% in patients treated with cerebral protection devices versus 5.5% in patients treated without cerebral protection devices. The death rates between the two groups showed no significant difference (0.8%, $P = 0.6$). However, these were primarily retrospective analyses of small studies and case series from single-center groups with no consistency in protection type (balloon versus filter), stent type, or operator experience. These possible confounding variables must be considered when the results of CAS procedures with cerebral protection devices are interpreted. Nevertheless, the authors concluded that in early analysis, the use of cerebral protection devices appeared to reduce thromboembolic complications during CAS. Ouriel et al. looked at a series of 261 patients who underwent CAS [3]. EPDs were used in 90 patients during this study. Debris in the retrieved filters was reported to be found in 54% of patients. There were fewer major ipsilateral strokes in the EPD group (0.0%) versus the group without EPDs (2.3%, $p = 0.05$). The authors concluded that EPDs may decrease the risk of postprocedural major ipsilateral strokes. Similarly, Cossotini et al. reported on their series of 52 patients who underwent CAS, 30 with EPD and 22 without EPD [4]. Magnetic resonance (MR) diffusion-weighted imaging (DWI) was performed in both groups of patients following stenting. Ischemic lesions were detected in 26% of patients in the protected group and 36% of patients in the unprotected group, with an overall incidence of 30% across both groups. In addition, the protected group was found to have fewer DWI lesions on MRI. There was no difference in the number of contralateral lesions between the two groups. These findings led to a recommendation that distal protection for carotid stenting may decrease the risk of ipsilateral stroke from CAS. As a result of some of the early evidence depicted by these studies, carotid stenting trials began to use EPDs in an effort to show equipoise to CEA. The Stenting and Angioplasty with Protection in Patients at High Risk for Endarterectomy (SAPPHIRE) trial mandated the use of EPDs in the stenting group in patients who were high risk for CEA [5]. The stroke or death rate within 30 days was 4.8% in patients treated with CAS versus 5.6% in CEA group. However, only a minority of the patients were randomized between stenting and carotid endarterectomy, and the enrollment in the CEA arm was very low in the nonrandomized group. In total, 334 patients were randomized, but 413 were not. Of this nonrandomized group, 406 had stenting with protection and only 7 had carotid endarterectomy. Therefore, instead of comparing outcomes to active controls, outcomes were compared to surgical and medical data in similar patient populations. Furthermore, the lower incidence of myocardial infarction (MI) in patients who underwent stenting may be attributed to the use of clopidogrel, which was not utilized in the CEA group. Interestingly, the lead author of SAPPHIRE invented the EPD used in the trial, and the majority of the remaining authors (11 of the 15) either worked for Cordis at the time or had financial relationships with the company [6]. Similarly, the ACCULINK for Revascularization of Carotids in High-Risk Patients (ARCHeR) trial reported that the 30-day death/stroke/myocardial infarction plus ipsilateral stroke at 1 year was 9.6% which is below the 14.4% reported in literature for CEA. The authors indicated that extracranial carotid artery stenting with embolic filter protection is noninferior to CEA [7]. As the SAPPHIRE and ARCHeR trials showed that CAS stenting with EPDs is noninferior to CEA, the trend of using EPDs in all future trials began. The Food and Drug Administration (FDA) consequently approved the ACCULINK stent and ACCUNET EPD based on data reported in the ARCHeR trial [8]. However, it should be noted that the FDA does not require use of EPDs with carotid stents. Nevertheless, EPDs are mandated for reimbursement by Medicare and used in more than 95% of all CAS cases in the United States. However, to date, no RCTs exist that compare protected and unprotected CAS with results depicting better outcomes with the use of EPDs.

The Evidence Against Distal Embolic Protection

The technical innovations in CAS are still ongoing and are aimed at increasing safety and decreasing complication rates. Theoretically, EPDs provide an effective mechanism to reduce periprocedural strokes during CAS. However, despite the results of several retrospective studies that support the use of EPDs, specifically distal protection devices (filters), some interventionalists are still concerned about the routine use of EPDs. The debate against the efficacy of EPDs during CAS rises from the fact that the risk of stroke associated with CAS is clearly related to embolic phenomena that occur during the intravascular instrumentation of the aortic arch, supra-aortic trunks, and carotid plaque itself. All these unprotected steps during the procedure are taken place before EPDs are installed. In addition, distal filters are bulky devices, and their use can be associated with internal carotid artery dissection, spasm, and embolic complications especially when tortuous anatomy and tight stenosis are present. The design also has important limitations as distal filters do not have ideal wall apposition, allowing material to embolize around the filter or particles smaller than their pore sizes to pass through. Furthermore, the filter can become overloaded with debris, thereby increasing the risk of dislodgement from the filter during recapturing. Additionally, recapturing and retrieving the filter can occasionally be difficult or fail, and filter contents can spill during this step as well. In this discussion, we aim to shed light on the results from the most recent prospective multicenter trials supporting the presumption that EPDs do not reduce but may actually increase CAS complication rates. Pro-CAS is a prospective registry of CAS procedures implemented by the German Society of Angiology/Vascular Medicine and the German Society of Radiology [9]. During the study's time frame, 4709 patients were included, 3543 of which were treated with EPDs and 1166 were treated without EPDs. Data analysis of the registry revealed no differences in periprocedural stroke or death rates between the two groups of patients (3.2% with EPDs vs. 3.4% without EPDs, $p = 0.6517$). These results are consistent with the Stent-Supported Percutaneous Angioplasty of the Carotid Artery versus Endarterectomy (SPACE) clinical trial that also assessed the use of EPDs in CAS procedures while also factoring in stent design (open vs. closed cell). Overall, 563 patients were treated with a stent, of which 145 patients were treated with EPDs and 418 without EPDs. Data analysis of patients that underwent CAS with and without EPDs showed that there was no difference in stroke or death rates between the two groups (8.3% vs. 6.2%, $p = 0.40$). When factoring in the stent design, there were significantly fewer adverse events in patients who underwent CAS with a closed-cell stent (5.5%), as opposed to those that were treated with an open stent (11%). Furthermore, there was no significant difference in adverse event rates with the use of EPDs in each stent design group: 6.7% in the closed-cell group versus 10% in the open-cell group ($p = 0.554$). When EPDs were not utilized, there was an adverse outcome rate of 5.3% in the closed-cell group vs. 12.3% in the open-cell group with no significant difference ($p = 0.068$) [10]. This secondary analysis of data does not support the need for EPDs in CAS. The Endarterectomy Versus Angioplasty in Patients with Symptomatic Carotid Stenosis (EVA-3S) trial assessed the utility of employing EPDs to modify the risk of periprocedural complications. After 80 patients were enrolled, the unprotected CAS arm was stopped early by the safety committee as the 30-day rate of stroke was 3.9 times higher than that of CAS with cerebral protection (4/15 vs. 5/58) [11]. However, the lower limits of the confidence interval indicated an absence of difference in adverse events between protected and unprotected CAS. In addition, most of the patients who underwent unprotected CAS and had an adverse event did so in the 30 days following the procedure and not during the procedure itself, thereby casting doubt on whether cerebral protection was truly a factor in inciting the adverse event. Another issue is the lack of randomization within the CAS group as to which patient undergoes the procedure with and without EPDs. The International Carotid Stenting Study (ICSS) looked at a subgroup of patients who underwent MRI before and after CAS and CEA. The CAS group was further subdivided into patients who underwent stenting with and without EPDs. Interestingly, more patients had new ischemic lesions on MRI diffusion-weighted imaging (DWI) after stenting with cerebral protection devices (37 of 51 (73%)) than without (25 of 73 (34%)) [12]. In addition, the rate of stroke was higher in the EPD group (5.1%) than the unprotected group (2.4%). The authors conclude that EPDs did not seem to be effective in preventing cerebral ischemia during stenting. Tietke and Jansen evaluated CAS with and without EPD by pooling data from multiple studies including SPACE, EVA-3S, and ICSS [13]. The authors concluded that the most recent data from multiple perspective multicenter trials support the impression that EPDs may actually increase the perioperative complication rates instead of reducing them. A couple of small, randomized trials also shed light on the postoperative events in CAS with and without EPDs. In one such study, Macdonald et al. showed that patients undergoing filter-protected CAS had significantly higher rates of total as well as particulate emboli on transcranial Doppler studies (426.5 and 251.3) than during unprotected CAS (165.2 and 92) ($p = 0.01$ and 0.03, respectively). On procedural MRI 1–3 hours and 24 hours after stenting, there was an increase in new lesions on DWI in 7/24 (29%) patients in the protected group and 4/22 (18%) patients in the unprotected group. At 30 days, lesions were detected in 9/33 (26%) patients in the protected group and in 4/33 (12%) patients in the unprotected group [14]. A small, randomized study by Barbato et al. showed similar results with new lesions noted on MRI in 72% of patients in the cerebral protection group and 44% of patients in the unprotected group ($p = 0.09$) [15]. In 2011, Tallarita et al. conducted a retrospective review of a prospective nonrandomized database at their institution of patients that underwent CAS with and without embolic protection [16]. They reviewed 357 CAS patients, 105 of whom underwent unprotected CAS and 252 of whom underwent filter-protected CAS. No significant difference in the primary end points of perioperative stroke rate (0.8% in the EP group vs. 3.8% in the non-EP group; $P = 0.6$), death (1 in each group), or MI (3 in the EP group and 1 in the non-EP group, P = nonsignificant) was discovered between the two groups. Similarly, Pandey et al. retrospectively reviewed a series of 105 patients that underwent CAS without the use of EPDs and reported a perioperative stroke and death rate of 2.85% [17]. The authors revealed that CAS can be performed safely, with similar risks and lower costs when compared to series in which EPDs were used. Interestingly, most patients in this study did not undergo post-stenting angioplasty. Pandey et al. showed that by avoiding this step, there were lower complication rates with unprotected CAS. However, the author did not discuss the significance of this nuance. Binning et al. retrospectively reviewed a data from our institute and reported a 0% perioperative stroke and death rate and 2% perioperative non-ST elevation myocardial infarction (NSTEMI) rate [18] in patients who underwent CAS without EPD and without post-stent plasty. In the CREST trial, the rate of minor stroke was 4.1%, rate of major stroke was 0.9%, and overall rate of stroke, death, and MI was 5.2% [1]. In our institution, the MI rate is 2%, which is comparable to the rate observed in the carotid endarterectomy (CEA) group from the CREST trial (2.3%) [1]. In addition, the rate of perioperative stroke and death rate in the SAPPHIRE trial was 3.6% [5]. The low rate observed in our group is most likely attributable to the fact that the majority of our cases are performed under general anesthesia. In general, our patient population is most comparable to the CREST trial patient population, as roughly 80% of our patients had symptomatic lesions, of which 75% were greater than 80% stenosed. In addition, a closed-cell design was used to treat our patients. Although we did not conduct post-stenting angioplasty, our restenosis rate requiring retreatment was only 2.8%, which is lower than the restenosis rate reported in the CREST trial where most patients underwent post-stenting angioplasty [1].

There are many steps involved in CAS, and each step carries the potential risk of embolic complications. Examples of such steps include crossing the lesions with wires, balloons and filters, pre- and post-stenting angioplasty, and stenting. Furthermore, when using open-cell stent designs, there is concern that plaque particles may pass through the stent pores, called the "cheese grater" effect. In the Carotid and Vertebral Artery Transluminal Angioplasty Study (CAVATAS) trial, most carotid procedures consisted of angioplasty only without stenting or without post-stenting angioplasty, thereby avoiding any associated embolic risks [19]. This might be why the results of the trial indicate that endovascular treatment is not inferior to CEA, despite the lack of distal protection. The low complication rates reported in this unprotected trial are of special interest since angioplasty alone is no longer recommended.

Overall, results from numerous single and multicenter studies indicate no difference in ischemic event rates with or without the use of embolic protection. On the other hand, these same studies report far lower adverse event rates in CAS without the use of EPDs when compared to large trials that incorporated the use of EPDs.

Innovations in distal EPDs may lead to improved outcomes, or studies might show compelling data suggesting that proximal protection is superior. To date, the potential utility of P-EPDs compared with F-EPDs has not been analyzed in large scale using the clinical outcomes of stroke and mortality. The most recent trials must also be juxtaposed with today's best medical therapy as well as CEA to truly identify the overall best management for carotid disease.

CREST-2 is an ongoing multicenter, randomized controlled trial, designed to compare three different methods of stroke prevention to find the safest and most effective treatment. It started in 2014 and planned to complete enrollment of 2480 patients by December 2022, but is still ongoing. The stroke prevention methods include intensive medical management alone compared to intensive medical management in combination with a CEA or CAS. The information from this study will help to refine the best individualized treatment approach for asymptomatic patients with carotid stenosis given modern interventional and medical management strategies.

Proximal Embolic Protection Devices and Transcarotid Artery Revascularization (TCAR)

Physicians who perform carotid interventions are well aware of the fact that CAS is associated with embolization risk. Multiple large randomized clinical trials have shown noninferiority of CAS compared to CEA when analyzing composite end points of myocardial infarction, stroke, and death. However, CAS has a higher risk of stroke within 30 days of intervention. In the CREST study, the periprocedural stroke rate was 4.1% vs. 2.3% for stenting vs. CEA, respectively. In contrast, midterm and long-term results show the risk of stroke beyond the operative period is similar and low between both treatment arms, respectively. Therefore, techniques to reduce the periprocedural stroke risk during stenting could make the two procedures equivalent across all time points. As the debate regarding the true efficacy of EPDs continues, proximal protection devices were developed to create flow arrest and even flow reversal during CAS procedures. Mokin et al. retrospectively reviewed a series of 70 patients who underwent CAS with proximal protection devices who were matched to another 70 cases treated with CAS with distal protection [20]. The authors reported no significant difference in 30-day adverse outcomes between the two groups ($P = 1.0$) even though there was a significantly higher number of high-risk lesions in proximal protection devices group ($P = 0.009$). Three additional small studies showed lower incidence (45.2% vs. 87.1%) and smaller volume of lesions (0.16 cm^3 vs. 0.59 cm^3) detected in MRI-DWI in patients who underwent proximal protection when compared to distal protection, but there was no difference in the number of adverse clinical or symptomatic events [21–23]. Flow reversal improves upon this idea. With advancements in technology and experience, transcarotid artery revascularization (TCAR) technique using the ENROUTE neuroprotection flow-reversal system was developed. This hybrid procedure combines the minimally invasive advantages of CAS while also using complete carotid artery blood flow reversal as neuroprotection. Briefly, the TCAR operation involves a small longitudinal or transverse skin incision at the base of the neck to access the CCA directly. The proximal common carotid artery (CCA) is exposed, and micropuncture needle, wire, and arterial sheath are used to obtain vascular access, obviating the need for unprotected catheter navigation of aortic or supra-aortic vessels. Simultaneously, the common femoral vein is percutaneously accessed, and the external circuit is completed, thereby initiating passive reversal of blood flow from the carotid artery. Before the intervention, the CCA is clamped proximal to the sheath, leading to obligatory carotid blood flow reversal. Flow reversal reduces the risk of embolism during all phases: lesion crossing, predilatation, stenting, and postdilatation. Proponents of the TCAR procedure argue that avoiding catheter manipulation in the aortic arch is important in decreasing the risks of periprocedural strokes from microemboli. However, there is some evidence that most microembolic infarcts demonstrated on MRI are not seen on the initial post-CAS MRI but appear on the 48-hour MRI, suggesting that the microemboli arise from the stent itself and not from catheter manipulation in the aortic arch [24]. Direct carotid access also has its own set of potential complications, similar to those seen in anterior cervical approaches in neurosurgery. For example, there is a risk of injury to the cranial nerves. However, because the cutdown is directed toward the common carotid artery, rather than the bifurcation, this risk of injury is decreased. Furthermore, the internal jugular vein is positioned adjacent to the carotid artery and could be injured during procedure. In addition, manipulation of the cervical muscles may cause swelling and postprocedural pain. Lastly, the development of a postprocedural hematoma could potentially compromise the airway.

The PROOF trial was the first-in-man study designed to evaluate the feasibility of this flow-reversal system [25]. It demonstrated new lesions on postprocedural DWI MRI in 5 of 31 patients (16%), although none of these patients experienced clinical sequelae. A larger, multicenter trial, Safety and Efficacy Study for Reverse Flow Used During Carotid Artery Stenting Procedure (ROADSTER), demonstrated success and efficacy in preventing stroke during CAS [26]. The device was successfully utilized in 99% of 141 patients enrolled in the study. The stroke rate was 1.4%, while the combined rate of stroke and death was 2.8%. However, among the symptomatic patients in this study, the authors did not mention how many patients had experienced symptoms recently (≤ 7 to 14 days before CAS) and how many patients experienced symptoms up to 6 months before CAS. Patients with recent symptoms would be expected to have a higher stroke rate than those with more distant symptoms. Additionally, there were eight carotid artery dissections associated with this device and one case of a severe common carotid artery stenosis caused by a purse-string suture. Kashyap VS et al. conducted a prospective, single-arm multicenter clinical trial to evaluate the 1-year safety and efficacy of TCAR [27]. One hundred fifty-five patients at 21 centers were enrolled. All patients were considered high risk for CEA. Over the year, no patient had an ipsilateral stroke, but four patients died (2.6%). None of the deaths were neurologic in origin. Additionally, a technical success rate of 98.7% with a low cranial nerve deficit rate of 1.3% was achieved. The authors concluded that TCAR offers a safe and durable revascularization option for patients who are deemed to be at high risk for CEA. However, this study is a single-arm clinical trial and lacks a control group. An RCT comparing the TCAR and ENROUTE NPS with CEA or TFCAS would be more rigorous in providing a noninferiority conclusion, and 1 year might not be reflective of the long-term beneficial impact of TCAR. Only long-term follow-up and further experience will tell us about the efficacy and potential complications of this device. In our institute, we offer a TCAR procedure to patients who are considered high risk for CEA and CAS, especially in cases of very tortuous and calcified aortic arches.

Conclusions

Treatment options for CAD are constantly evolving. Many single and multicenter studies previously described in this chapter show clear evidence that the use of embolic protection devices does not enhance the safety of CAS. Additionally, multiple studies show no difference in outcomes between protected and unprotected CAS, regardless of if protection is used distally or proximally. Moreover, some larger registries and trials actually show worse outcomes with the use of distal EPDs. Present distal filters are unlikely to be the final solution in making CAS as safe as possible. With advancements in technology and experience, reflected by improved outcomes in prospective RCTs, the indications, applications, and safety of CAS will expand.

The use of distal filter EPDs for CAS has been handed down as a directive despite the lack of adequate evidence portraying their benefits and efficacy. Overall, there is uncertainty regarding the efficacy of EPDs in preventing thromboembolic complications during CAS procedures. However, a new and appealing procedure or device must always be tested and its efficacy clearly proven across multiple scenarios before recommending its use. Successful implementation of such techniques or devices in certain situations by certain skilled operators does not make them generalizable to other groups. Despite all this, many institutions and multiple studies have shown that unprotected CAS can indeed be performed safely and effectively. The present "standard" to perform CAS with EPDs should be further scrutinized with RCTs, and the results from these trials should then dictate the use of EPDs. Until then, distal filter-protected CAS should be considered when appropriate and utilized cautiously at the operator's discretion.

References

1. Mantese VA, Timaran CH, Chiu D, Begg RJ, Brott TG, CREST investigators. The Carotid Revascularization Endarterectomy Versus Stenting Trial (CREST) stenting versus carotid endarterectomy for carotid disease. Stroke. 2010;41:S31–4.
2. Kastrup A, Gröschel K, Krapf H, Brehm BR, Dichgans J, Schulz JB. Early outcome of carotid angioplasty and stenting with and without cerebral protection devices: a systematic review of the literature. Stroke. 2003;34:813–9.
3. Ouriel K, Wholey MH, Fayad P, Katzen BT, Whitlow P, Frentzko M, et al. Feasibility trial of carotid stenting with and without an embolus protection device. J Endovasc Ther. 2005;12:525–37.
4. Cosottini M, Michelassi MC, Puglioli M, Lazzarotti G, Orlandi G, Marconi F, et al. Silent cerebral ischemia detected with diffusion-weighted imaging in patients treated with protected and unprotected carotid artery stenting. Stroke. 2005;36:2389–93.
5. Yadav JS, Wholey MH, Kuntz RE, Fayad P, Katzen BT, Mishkel GJ, Stenting and Angioplasty with Protection in Patients at High Risk for Endarterectomy Investigators, et al. Protected carotid-artery stenting versus endarterectomy in high risk patients. N Engl J Med. 2004;351:1493–501.
6. Thomas DJ. Protected carotid artery stenting versus endarterectomy in high-risk patients: reflections from SAPPHIRE. Stroke. 2005;36:912–3.
7. Gray WA, Hopkins LN, Yadav S, Davis T, Wholey M, Atkinson R, ARCHeR Trial Collaborators, et al. Protected carotid stenting in high-surgical-risk patients: the ARCHeR results. J Vasc Surg. 2006;44:258–68.
8. Toor SA, Cavanaugh KJ, Lim LM. Regulation of carotid artery stents and embolic protection devices in the United States. A history of, and perspectives on, FDA regulation of carotid stents and associated embolic protection devices over the years. Endovasc Today. 2013:44–58.
9. Theiss W, Hermanek P, Mathias K, Bruckmann H, Dembski J, Hoffmann FJ, et al. Predictors of death and stroke after carotid angioplasty and stenting: a subgroup analysis of the PRO-CAS data. Stroke. 2008;39:2325–30.
10. Jansen O, Fiehler J, Hartmann M, Bruckmann H. Protection or nonprotection in carotid stent angioplasty the influence of interventional techniques on outcome data from the SPACE trial. Stroke. 2009;40:841–6.
11. EVA-3S Investigators. Carotid angioplasty and stenting with and without cerebral protection clinical alert from the endarterectomy versus angioplasty in patients with symptomatic severe carotid stenosis (EVA-3S) trial. Stroke. 2004;35:e18–21.

12. Bonati LH, Jongen LM, Haller S, Flach HZ, Dobson J, Nederkoorn PJ, ICSS-MRI Study Group. New ischaemic brain lesions on MRI after stenting or endarterectomy for symptomatic carotid stenosis: a substudy of the International Carotid Stenting Study (ICSS). Lancet Neurol. 2010;9(4):353–62.

13. Tietke M, Jansen O. Cerebral protection vs no cerebral protection: timing of stroke with CAS. J Cardiovasc Surg. 2009;50(6):751–60.

14. Macdonald S, Evans DH, Griffiths PD, et al. Filter-protected versus unprotected carotid artery stenting: a randomised trial. Cerebrovasc Dis. 2010;29:282–9.

15. Barbato JE, Dillavou E, Horowitz MB, et al. A randomized trial of carotid artery stenting with and without cerebral protection. J Vasc Surg. 2008;47:760–5.

16. Tallarita T, Rabinstein AA, Cloft H, et al. Are distal protection devices 'protective' during carotid angioplasty and stenting? Stroke. 2011;42:1962–6.

17. Pandey AS, Koebbe CJ, Liebman K, Rosenwasser RH, Veznedaroglu E. Low incidence of symptomatic strokes after carotid stenting without embolization protection devices for extracranial carotid stenosis: a single-institution retrospective review. Neurosurgery. 2008;63:867–73.

18. Binning MJ, Maxwell CR, Stofko D, Zerr M, Maghazehe K, Liebman K, Hakma Z, Lewis-Diaz C, Veznedaroglu E. Carotid artery angioplasty and stenting without distal embolic protection devices. Neurosurgery. 2017;80(1):60–4. https://doi.org/10.1227/NEU.0000000000001367. PMID: 27471973.

19. Endovascular versus surgical treatment in patients with carotid stenosis in the Carotid and Vertebral Transluminal Angioplasty Study (CAVATAS): a randomised trial. Lancet. 2001;357:1729–37.

20. Mokin M, Dumont TM, Chi JM, Manhan CJ, Kass-Hout T, Sorkin G, et al. Proximal versus distal protection during carotid artery stenting: analysis of the two treatment approaches and associated clinical outcomes. World Neurosurg. 2014;81(3/4):543–8.

21. Leal I, Orgaz A, Flores A, Gil J, Rodriguez R, Peinado J, et al. A diffusion-weighted magnetic resonance imaging-based study of transcervical carotid stenting with flow reversal vs transfemoral filter protection. J Vasc Surg. 2012;56:1585–90.

22. Bijuklic K, Wandler A, Hazizi F, Schofer J. The PROFI study (prevention of cerebral embolization by proximal balloon occlusion compared to filter protection during carotid artery stenting): a prospective randomized trial. J Am Coll Cardiol. 2012;59:1383–9.

23. Cano MN, Kambara AM, de Cano SJF, Portela LAP, Paes AT, Costa JR. Randomized comparison of distal and proximal cerebral protection during carotid artery stenting. J Am Coll Cardiol Intv. 2013;6:1204–9.

24. Rapp JH, Wakil L, Sawhney R, Pan XM, Yenari MA, Glastonbury C, Coogan S, Wintermark M. Subclinical embolization after carotid artery stenting: new lesions on diffusion-weighted magnetic resonance imaging occur postprocedure. J Vasc Surg. 2007;45(5):867–72; discussion 872-4. https://doi.org/10.1016/j.jvs.2006.12.058. Epub 2007 Mar 21. PMID: 17376643.

25. Pinter L, Ribo M, Loh C, Lane B, Roberts T, Chou TM, Kolvenbach RR. Safety and feasibility of a novel transcervical access neuroprotection system for carotid artery stenting in the PROOF study. J Vasc Surg. 2011;54(5):1317–23. https://doi.org/10.1016/j.jvs.2011.04.040. Epub 2011 Jun 12. PMID: 21658889.

26. Kwolek CJ, Jaff MR, Leal JI, Hopkins LN, Shah RM, Hanover TM, Macdonald S, Cambria RP. Results of the ROADSTER multicenter trial of transcarotid stenting with dynamic flow reversal. J Vasc Surg. 2015;62(5):1227–34. https://doi.org/10.1016/j.jvs.2015.04.460. PMID: 26506270.

27. Kashyap VS, So KL, Schneider PA, Rathore R, Pham T, Motaganahalli RL, Massop DW, Foteh MI, Eckstein HH, Jim J, Leal Lorenzo JI, Melton JG. One-year outcomes after Transcarotid Artery Revascularization (TCAR) in the ROADSTER 2 TRIAL. J Vasc Surg. 2022:S0741-5214(22)01366-0. https://doi.org/10.1016/j.jvs.2022.03.872. Epub ahead of print. PMID: 35381327.

Closing the Gap: Addressing the Lag in Stroke Care Evolution

6

Erol Veznedaroglu, Karen Greenberg, and Haley Fitzgerald

Introduction

The management of acute ischemic stroke (AIS) has evolved, albeit very slowly, since the first use of tissue plasminogen activator (tPA) in 1996 after receiving FDA approval. The early adaptation was rocky as many emergency providers were the first line, and a serious complication was intracerebral hemorrhage. The original National Institute of Neurological Disorders of Stroke

E. Veznedaroglu (✉)
Department of Neurosurgery, Drexel University School of Medicine, Philadelphia, PA, USA

Global Neurosciences Institute, Pennington, NJ, USA
e-mail: evez@gnineuro.org

K. Greenberg
Departments of Clinical Education, Emergency Medicine, Neurosurgery, Drexel University School of Medicine, Philadelphia, PA, USA

Department of Neurology, Temple Lewis Katz School of Medicine, Philadelphia, PA, USA

H. Fitzgerald
Department of Neurosurgery, Global Neurosciences Institute, Pennington, NJ, USA
e-mail: hfitzgerald@gnineuro.org

© The Author(s), under exclusive license to Springer Nature Switzerland AG 2025
E. Veznedaroglu (ed.), *Advanced Technologies in Vascular Neurosurgery*, https://doi.org/10.1007/978-3-031-67492-1_6

(NINDS) data was conflicting and primarily based on animal models [1–6]. The first pilot study was conducted in 1992, with a 90-minute time window [7]. Subsequent pilot studies looked at dose escalation and timing window, with phase 2 trials extending to 180 minutes [8]. Ultimately, intravenous (IV) tPA was approved and accepted as the standard of care for AIS for up to 3 hours and extended to 4.5 hours in 2009 [9]. In context, animal data from the early 1990s led to the commencement of the first clinical trials in only several years (1995). Thus, our "starting point" of giving IV tPA to patients suffering from AIS was three decades ago.

Despite progress in intra-arterial treatments, including extending time windows and better use of imaging, IV thrombolytic therapy has been stagnant. The use of perfusion imaging to extend treatment and better understand patient selection has driven this progress. Unfortunately, IV treatments have not progressed with the same modalities. This is concerning because IV thrombolytics are the "first line" and most readily available at most centers in the emergency department setting. Perfusion imaging has allowed extended treatments in Europe and will likely show better outcomes by better patient selection [10]. The treatment paradigm for AIS has lagged behind almost every other emergent condition.

Trauma has had rigorous guidelines with frequent updates based on best practices. The designation of a dedicated center for traumatic injuries is clearly defined for both communities and emergency medical services (EMS). Lifesaving triage is the cornerstone of both emergent transport and ensuring appropriate resources and personnel at designated trauma centers. Evidence that the organization of cardiovascular care may be effective in reducing morbidity and mortality has existed since at least the 1950s when cardiologists implemented specialized care in coronary units for patients with acute heart disease [11]. Comprehensive stroke centers have emerged more recently, and it took even longer to establish a "hub and spoke" model. The first certification process for a primary stroke center was 20 years ago, in 2004 [12].

Emergency physicians will give tPA for coronary events routinely. However, it is rare for them to provide IV thrombolytics for AIS. The reliance on a "specialist" to be consulted to approve its delivery delays care that is time sensitive. This is even more alarming given that, in 2020, 1 in 21 deaths in the United States was due to stroke. Even more sobering is the fact that every 3 minutes, someone in the United States will die of a stroke [13]. Few would argue that present treatments and paradigms have been too slow to be adopted. Newer models and outdated practices should be reconsidered, considering the journey of thrombolytics from mouse to man. We will discuss several concepts and practices that have already begun to emerge and hopefully will lead to better care of the AIS patient.

Specialized Neurologic Emergency Departments

The primary catalyst for innovation in the provision of care to AIS patients lies in the establishment of a dedicated neurologic emergency department (neuro ED). While specialized emergency departments (EDs), such as those for pediatrics, have been in operation since 1989, the replication of similar programs targeting different age groups (geriatrics) or specific diseases (ST-elevation myocardial infarction, trauma) has demonstrated enhanced cost-effectiveness and, ultimately, improved patient outcomes [14–16]. Despite substantial advancements in the diagnosis and treatment of neurological and neurosurgical emergencies, the training of emergency department physicians and the integration of hospital resources in this domain, especially in stroke treatment, have lagged behind [17].

Since 2011, two dedicated neuro EDs have been established in New Jersey and Pennsylvania. These specialized areas within the main ED are staffed by board-certified emergency medicine physicians with additional neurological education. The training can encompass rotations through the neurologic intensive care unit, specialized stroke unit, and neuro-interventional operating room. Physicians also have the option to engage in one-on-one sessions with fellowship-trained neuroradiologists for the interpretation of neurological imaging studies. Alternative avenues for acquiring neurological education include participation in neurologic continuing medical education courses and attendance at neuroscience conferences to augment knowledge and skill sets [18].

The neuro ED is equipped with comprehensive imaging resources, including computed tomography (CT) scan, CT angiography (CTA), CT perfusion (CTP), magnetic resonance imaging (MRI), magnetic resonance angiography, and electroencephalogram. The allocation of a dedicated section within the ED for identifying, triaging, and treating patients with neurological emergencies results in more advanced and efficient care, minimizing unnecessary studies and tests that may cause delays in therapeutic treatments. A retrospective observational study conducted from 2019 to 2021 compared outcomes of acute ischemic stroke patients treated in the neuro ED and a traditional emergency department (TED). The analysis revealed significant reductions in door-to-needle times (DTN) and door-to-CT times (DTCT) in the neuro ED [19] (Table 6.1). The evidence unequivocally supports the notion that acute stroke patients receive faster diagnostics and treatment in a dedicated neuro ED.

However, time is just one facet of stroke algorithms; it must translate into improved outcomes. While the admission National Institutes of Health Stroke Scale (NIHSS) showed a nonsignificant difference, the discharge NIHSS demonstrated a statistically significant reduction in the neuro ED [19]. Furthermore, a significantly higher proportion of patients could be discharged to their homes after hospitalization if care originated in the neuro ED compared to the TED [18]. These findings underscore the

Table 6.1 Neuro ED vs. traditional ED

	Neuro ED	Traditional ED	p-value
Number of patients treated 2019–2021	74	45	
Average door-to-needle time	27 minutes	65 minutes	$p < 0.001$
Average door-to-CT time	13 minutes	22 minutes	$p < 0.001$
Admission NIHSS	8.1	9.4	$p = 0.17$
Discharge NIHSS	2.4	5.6	$p = 0.001$

Retrospective observational study from 2019 to 2021 comparing outcomes of acute ischemic stroke patients who received IV alteplase following implementation of the neuro ED compared to a traditional emergency department (TED)

transformative impact of a dedicated neuro ED on expediting care, enhancing efficiency, and ultimately improving patient outcomes in acute ischemic stroke.

The core clinical privileges in emergency medicine encompass the administration of thrombolytic therapy for myocardial infarction and stroke. Traditionally, emergency medicine providers have relied on neurology specialty consultation to treat acute stroke patients. However, the neurologic emergency department (neuro ED) introduces a groundbreaking paradigm where emergency medicine physicians independently assess and administer intravenous (IV) alteplase or tenecteplase to acute ischemic stroke (AIS) patients without the need for teleneurology or specialty consultation.

The Target: Stroke initiative, led by the American Heart Association/American Stroke Association, has enhanced stroke outcomes by reducing door-to-needle times for eligible ischemic stroke patients [20]. Phase III of this initiative raises the standard by setting more ambitious targets for timely treatment with IV thrombolytics (IVT). The primary goal is to achieve door-to-needle times within 60 minutes in 85% or more of AIS patients treated with IVT. Secondary goals include achieving door-to-needle times within 45 minutes in 75% or more of AIS patients and within 30 minutes in 50% or more of AIS patients [20].

Despite the well-documented benefits of IV alteplase and the recommendation for rapid administration, the delivery remains suboptimal, with approximately 53.3% of eligible patients in the United States receiving treatment within the recommended time window [21]. The delay in administering IV alteplase is attributed to various factors, with a significant contributor being the timing between symptom onset and the decision to administer the medication, often made through teleneurology or neurologist consultation in many medical centers.

The implementation of a neuro ED has transformed this landscape, empowering emergency medicine physicians to independently and safely administer IVT. This autonomy has resulted in significantly reduced door-to-needle (DTN) times, lower National Institutes of Health Stroke Scale (NIHSS) scores on discharge, and a higher likelihood of patients being discharged to their homes compared to subacute rehabilitation or extended care facilities, as discussed earlier. The neuro ED aligns with the goals of Target: Stroke Phase III and represents a pioneering approach that addresses the multifactorial challenges in timely stroke treatment, ultimately improving patient outcomes and quality of care.

The Emergency Medicine Provider as a "Stroke Champion"

An innovative feature of the neuro ED is the designation of physicians as stroke champions (SCs). The 2013 American Academy of Neurology study revealed an 11% shortage of neurologists, projected to increase to 19% by 2025, with a demand for 3000 additional neurologists [22]. To address this global shortage, teleneurology and telestroke care have been implemented, particularly for AIS patients. SCs, as mentioned earlier, autonomously treat AIS patients with fibrinolytic therapy and provide teleneurology to fellow emergency physicians at spoke hospitals, offering a novel solution to the ongoing shortage.

SCs operate from the hub hospital, functioning as a command center equipped with a dedicated smartphone for stroke calls from spoke hospitals. Communication occurs primarily over the phone, with an option for video evaluation, utilizing a shared picture archiving and communication system (PACS) for immediate neuroimage review. SCs can consult a vascular neurosurgeon and general neurologist directly through a hotline if needed, ensuring swift decision-making and avoiding delays in patient care [23].

In a retrospective study spanning 19 months, the neuro ED's command center received 457 phone calls for patients meeting stroke alert criteria. SCs managed blood pressure, dosed thrombolytics, and provided recommendations for advanced neuroimaging. They extensively reviewed inclusion and exclusion criteria for IVT with spoke emergency physicians and facilitated transfers for eligible patients. The study reported a 6.25% incidence of symptomatic intracranial hemorrhage (sICH) for patients receiving IV thrombolytics, consistent with the National Institute of Neurological Disorders and Stroke (NINDS) trial [24].

While concerns about intracranial hemorrhage post-thrombolytic administration persist, it is noteworthy that patients are more likely to sue physicians for not administering thrombolytics promptly [25]. The neuro ED model, with its emphasis on SCs, can be generalized to empower all emergency physicians to confidently administer thrombolytics to AIS patients, thereby improving outcomes and delivering optimal patient care. This innovative approach addresses the shortage of neurologists and sets a precedent for advancing stroke care within emergency medicine.

Extending the IV Thrombolytic Window

The treatment rates for stroke in the United States have persistently remained at notably low levels over several decades. Large-vessel occlusion, a condition affecting only an estimated 10–30% of all patients with AIS, underscores the continued significance of IVT as the primary therapeutic approach [26]. Most AIS patients are ineligible for endovascular therapy (EVT), emphasizing the continued importance of IVT in the treatment paradigm.

Despite the Food and Drug Administration (FDA) approving thrombolytics for acute ischemic stroke in 1996, their utilization in the United States has not witnessed a commensurate increase. Notably, from 2007 (2.8%) to 2014 (7.7%), the usage of IVT has experienced a modest rise [27]. However, a substantial proportion of eligible patients remains untreated, indicative of an unmet need within the present healthcare landscape. One primary contributing factor to the suboptimal administration of IVT is the constrained time window, requiring patients to present within 4.5 hours of their last known well status to initiate treatment.

The landscape of AIS treatment is undergoing rapid transformation, driven by advancements in neuroimaging and a shift from reliance on time windows to tissue windows. The WAKEUP and MR WITNESS studies have demonstrated the feasibility of treating patients beyond a definitive last known well time, challenging the conventional temporal constraints of stroke intervention. However, a notable limitation of both studies lies in their reliance on magnetic resonance imaging (MRI) for advanced neuroimaging, a resource not ubiquitously available in many emergency departments across the United States. Furthermore, certain medical conditions, such as the presence of pacemakers, spinal stimulators, retained foreign bodies, or claustrophobia, preclude the use of MRI in some stroke patients.

Addressing these challenges, the EXTEND trial, published in 2019, investigated the applicability of IVT guided by CT perfusion imaging up to 9 hours poststroke onset [28]. This trial focused on patients with ischemic stroke who exhibited hypoperfused but salvageable brain regions as detected by automated perfusion imaging. More of the alteplase-treated patients achieved a favorable outcome (modified Rankin Scale score 0–1) compared to the control group, with rates of symptomatic intracerebral hemorrhage similar to the original NINDS trial [24]. The use of CT perfusion imaging overcomes practical limitations associated with MRI accessibility and establishes a more universally applicable model for emergency departments (EDs) throughout the United States. The findings from the EXTEND trial contribute valuable insights into the potential expansion of the treatment window for acute ischemic stroke patients, offering a pragmatic and feasible alternative for EDs in the United States.

To further substantiate the use of IVT guided by perfusion imaging within a 9-hour window, our group has initiated patient enrollment in a trial modeled after the EXTEND trial. Our study similarly uses the modified Rankin Scale to measure improvement after 90 days and measures symptomatic intracerebral hemorrhage as a secondary outcome. There is presently a cohort of five patients showing promising results. If additional trials affirm the safety and efficacy of this extended treatment, stroke protocols may evolve to preserve more salvageable brain tissue in patients with AIS.

Tenecteplase: A Promising Alternative to Alteplase in AIS Management

The WAKEUP, MR WITNESS, and EXTEND trials conducted in recent years have prominently featured alteplase as the primary thrombolytic agent for the treatment of ischemic stroke. Despite its long-standing use spanning over two decades, alteplase, owing to its limited recanalization efficacy and associated risk of intracerebral hemorrhage, has prompted considerations regarding its suitability as the optimal thrombolytic drug.

A promising alternative is tenecteplase (TNK), a genetically engineered mutant tissue plasminogen activator exhibiting pharmacokinetic advantages such as enhanced fibrin selectivity and an extended half-life [29]. TNK presents several advantages over alteplase, including simplified dosing calculations, a single bolus administration, and logistical ease of transport between hospital systems, eliminating the need for continuous infusion.

Several trials within the past few years have explored the safety and efficacy of extending the treatment window using TNK as the primary thrombolytic in stroke management. In 2022, the CHABLIS-T trial in China examined the use of TNK up to 24 hours after the onset of AIS caused by large-vessel occlusions with significant penumbral mismatch on perfusion CT [30]. The trial's findings indicated that the lower dose of tenecteplase (0.25 mg/kg) yielded a higher rate of major reperfusion without symptomatic hemorrhage, albeit with a lower likelihood of excellent neurological outcomes compared to the higher dose (27.9% vs. 48.8%) [30].

More recently, trials like ROSE-TNK, TWIST, and TIMELESS have explored the efficacy and safety of TNK in various settings, reflecting a paradigm shift toward its extended use beyond conventional time windows [31–33]. These studies have further shown neurological improvement in the acute phase of AIS [34]. The use of non-contrast CT in TWIST is particularly significant as it suggests a translatable model to most emergency departments (EDs) nationwide, where advanced neuroimaging resources may be limited. TIMELESS and ROSE-TNK shed light on the potential time constraints of TNK's present use [31, 32]. Notably, TNK exhibited higher odds of complete recanalization in patients undergoing mechanical thrombectomy, suggesting a possible synergistic effect when employed in conjunction with endovascular interventions [34].

Given the limited eligibility for endovascular thrombectomy (EVT) in a small percentage of AIS patients, there is a compelling need to explore and expand the boundaries of IVT utilization.

Shifting focus from rigid time windows to assessing tissue windows through advanced neuroimaging remains crucial. Ongoing randomized controlled trials in this field, supported by the evolving evidence surrounding TNK, hold the promise of broadening treatment opportunities for acute ischemic stroke patients. Continued efforts in this direction are pivotal for advancing the field and improving outcomes for individuals affected by ischemic stroke.

Neuroprotectives in Post-thrombectomy Ischemic Stroke Recovery

Although much attention has been paid to the efficacy of intra-arterial thrombectomy over the past decade [35], little has been done to assess cell recovery after stroke. This is surprising given the fact that we have a direct route and access to the penumbra region after every successful thrombectomy. A micro-catheter is positioned in the vessel previously occluded with direct distribution to anoxic parenchyma. Emerging studies have explored different medications to counteract detrimental molecular events in conjunction with accepted strategies to restore blood flow for optimal recovery [36]. Despite these efforts, the use of any of these agents has yet to become universally accepted.

Our group sought to determine the safety of injecting 10 mg of verapamil after a successful thrombectomy in the region of the ischemic penumbra. Verapamil was chosen as it is known for its suspected neuroprotective properties in animal models [37, 38]. Also, it is widely used in neurointervention for the treatment of vasospasm and is tolerated exceptionally well [39]. Our initial data showed statistically significant improvement in mRS scores in 20 patients age-matched with 23 placebo patients. Intra-arterial verapamil treatment was associated with significant decreases in mRS score, improved recovery time, and shortened length of hospital stay compared to standard-of-care treatment. This study suggests that verapamil is a safe and effective neuroprotective drug in clinical populations who experience an ischemic stroke and require mechanical thrombectomy [40].

Conclusion

Stroke treatment has progressed slowly despite the considerable attention it now receives. Organizations such as the American Heart Association (AHA) have been primarily focused on heart disease, with stroke being a recent initiative. Multiple poorly designed studies in well-respected journals essentially halted the care of acute stroke patients for years with poor study designs and lack of understanding of treatments [41–43]. Not until MRCLEAN and DAWN trials did we understand the need for advancements in the treatment of AIS and the potential for surgical and medical intervention [35, 44]. This underscored the importance of treating stroke as a true emergency, similar to trauma and ST-elevation myocardial infarction (STEMI).

Since the publication of these studies, improved triage and a better understanding of the benefits of timely intervention have advanced stroke care and improved outcomes of patients [45]. As we look to the next decade of AIS, including prevention, post-acute care, and treatment options for those already affected by ischemic and hemorrhagic disease, we need to use all the tools available to us. This includes artificial intelligence (AI), virtual reality (VR), and advanced neuroimaging to implement functional neurosurgery. For the first time in history, technology has outpaced our ability to understand its best use. We must be vigilant as providers to break down traditional thinking and paradigms to "think outside the box" to help our patients better.

References

1. Zivin JA, Fisher M, DeGirolami U, Hemenway CC, Stashak JA. Tissue plasminogen activator reduces neurological damage after cerebral embolism. Science. 1985;230(4731):1289–92.
2. Penar PL, Greer CA. The effect of intravenous tissue-type plasminogen activator in a rat model of embolic cerebral ischemia. Yale J Biol Med. 1987;60(3):233–43.
3. Zivin JA, Lyden PD, DeGirolami U, Kochhar A, Mazzarella V, Hemenway CC, et al. Tissue plasminogen activator. Reduction of neurologic damage after experimental embolic stroke. Arch Neurol. 1988;45(4):387–91.

4. Phillips DA, Fisher M, Smith TW, Davis MA. The safety and angiographic efficacy of tissue plasminogen activator in a cerebral embolization model. Ann Neurol. 1988;23(4):391–4.

5. Lyden PD, Zivin JA, Clark WA, Madden K, Sasse KC, Mazzarella VA, et al. Tissue plasminogen activator-mediated thrombolysis of cerebral emboli and its effect on hemorrhagic infarction in rabbits. Neurology. 1989;39(5):703–8.

6. Overgaard K, Sereghy T, Boysen G, Pedersen H, Diemer NH. Reduction of infarct volume and mortality by thrombolysis in a rat embolic stroke model. Stroke. 1992;23(8):1167–73; discussion 1174

7. Brott TG, Haley EC, Levy DE, Barsan W, Broderick J, Sheppard GL, et al. Urgent therapy for stroke. Part I. Pilot study of tissue plasminogen activator administered within 90 minutes. Stroke. 1992;23(5):632–40.

8. Haley EC, Levy DE, Brott TG, Sheppard GL, Wong MC, Kongable GL, et al. Urgent therapy for stroke. Part II. Pilot study of tissue plasminogen activator administered 91-180 minutes from onset. Stroke. 1992;23(5):641–5.

9. Del Zoppo GJ, Saver JL, Jauch EC, Adams HP, American Heart Association Stroke Council. Expansion of the time window for treatment of acute ischemic stroke with intravenous tissue plasminogen activator: a science advisory from the American Heart Association/American Stroke Association. Stroke. 2009;40(8):2945–8.

10. Campbell BCV, Ma H, Ringleb PA, Parsons MW, Churilov L, Bendszus M, et al. Extending thrombolysis to 4·5-9 h and wake-up stroke using perfusion imaging: a systematic review and meta-analysis of individual patient data. Lancet. 2019;394(10193):139–47.

11. Julian DG. The evolution of the coronary care unit. Cardiovasc Res. 2001;51(4):621–4.

12. Gorelick PB. Primary and comprehensive stroke centers: history, value and certification criteria. J Stroke. 2013;15(2):78–89.

13. Tsao CW, Aday AW, Almarzooq ZI, Anderson CAM, Arora P, Avery CL, et al. Heart disease and stroke statistics-2023 update: a report from the American Heart Association. Circulation. 2023;147(8):e93–621.

14. Li M, Baker MD, Ropp LJ. Pediatric emergency medicine: a developing subspecialty. Pediatrics. 1989;84(2):336–42.

15. American College of Emergency Physicians, American Geriatrics Society, Emergency Nurses Association, Society for Academic Emergency Medicine, Geriatric Emergency Department Guidelines Task Force. Geriatric emergency department guidelines. Ann Emerg Med. 2014;63(5):e7–25.

16. Cooper C, Militello P. The multi-injured patient: the Maryland shock trauma protocol approach. Semin Thorac Cardiovasc Surg. 1992;4(3):163–7.

17. Veznedaroglu E, Rubin M, D'Ambrosio M. The neurological emergency room: the future is here. World Neurosurg. 2011;75(3–4):341–3.

18. Greenberg K, Maxwell CR, Moore KD, D'Ambrosio M, Liebman K, Veznedaroglu E, et al. Improved door-to-needle times and neurologic outcomes when IV tissue plasminogen activator is administered by emergency physicians with advanced neuroscience training. Am J Emerg Med. 2015;33(2):234–7.
19. Greenberg K, Bathini A, Maxwell C, Binning M, Veznedaroglu E. Improved patient outcomes in a specialized neurological emergency department. Moderated poster presentation at: International Stroke Conference; 2022; New Orleans, LA. Published in: Stroke. 2022;53(Suppl_1).
20. www.heart.org [Internet]. [cited 2024 Mar 26]. Target: stroke phase III. Available from: https://www.heart.org/en/professional/quality-improvement/target-stroke/introducing-target-stroke-phase-iii.
21. Ormseth CH, Sheth KN, Saver JL, Fonarow GC, Schwamm LH. The American Heart Association's Get With the Guidelines (GWTG)-stroke development and impact on stroke care. Stroke Vasc Neurol. 2017;2(2):94–105.
22. Dall TM, Storm MV, Chakrabarti R, Drogan O, Keran CM, Donofrio PD, et al. Supply and demand analysis of the current and future US neurology workforce. Neurology. 2013;81(5):470–8.
23. Greenberg K, Veznedaroglu E, Liebman K, Hakma Z, Kurtz T, Binning M. Stroke thrombolysis given by emergency physicians: the time is here. Am J Emerg Med. 2023;68:98–101.
24. National Institute of Neurological Disorders and Stroke rt-PA Stroke Study Group. Tissue plasminogen activator for acute ischemic stroke. N Engl J Med. 1995;333(24):1581–8.
25. Kwon B, George A, Plamoottil C, Stead T, Ganti L. 119 acute stroke, thrombolytics and litigation: reasons physicians get sued. Ann Emerg Med. 2021;78:S48–9.
26. Rocha M, Jovin TG. Fast versus slow progressors of infarct growth in large vessel occlusion stroke. Stroke. 2017;48(9):2621–7.
27. Meng T, Trickey AW, Harris AHS, Matheson L, Rosenthal S, Traboulsi AAR, et al. Lessons learned from the historical trends on thrombolysis use for acute ischemic stroke among medicare beneficiaries in the United States. Front Neurol. 2022;13:827965.
28. Ma H, Campbell BCV, Parsons MW, Churilov L, Levi CR, Hsu C, et al. Thrombolysis guided by perfusion imaging up to 9 hours after onset of stroke. N Engl J Med. 2019;380(19):1795–803.
29. Li G, Wang C, Wang S, Xiong Y, Zhao X. Tenecteplase in ischemic stroke: challenge and opportunity. Neuropsychiatr Dis Treat. 2022;18:1013–26.
30. Cheng X. Tenecteplase thrombolysis for stroke up to 24 hours after onset with perfusion imaging selection. Stroke Vasc Neurol. 2024:svn-2023-002820.

31. Wang L, Dai YJ, Cui Y, Zhang H, Jiang CH, Duan YJ, et al. Intravenous Tenecteplase for acute ischemic stroke within 4.5–24 hours of onset (ROSE-TNK): a phase 2, randomized, multicenter study. J Stroke. 2023;25(3):371–7.

32. Albers GW, Mouhammad J, Barbara P, Zaidi SF, Christopher S, Ashfaq S, et al. Tenecteplase for stroke at 4.5 to 24 hours with perfusion-imaging selection. N Engl J Med. 2024;390(8):701–11.

33. Roaldsen MB, Eltoft A, Wilsgaard T, Christensen H, Engelter ST, Indredavik B, et al. Safety and efficacy of tenecteplase in patients with wake-up stroke assessed by non-contrast CT (TWIST): a multicentre, open-label, randomised controlled trial. Lancet Neurol. 2023;22(2):117–26.

34. Palaiodimou L, Katsanos AH, Turc G, Romoli M, Theodorou A, Lemmens R, et al. Tenecteplase for the treatment of acute ischemic stroke in the extended time window: a systematic review and meta-analysis. Ther Adv Neurol Disord. 2024;17:17562864231221324.

35. Nogueira RG, Jadhav AP, Haussen DC, Bonafe A, Budzik RF, Bhuva P, et al. Thrombectomy 6 to 24 hours after stroke with a mismatch between deficit and infarct. N Engl J Med. 2018;378(1):11–21.

36. Paul S, Candelario-Jalil E. Emerging neuroprotective strategies for the treatment of ischemic stroke: an overview of clinical and preclinical studies. Exp Neurol. 2021;335:113518.

37. Maniskas ME, Roberts JM, Aron I, Fraser JF, Bix GJ. Stroke neuroprotection revisited: intra-arterial verapamil is profoundly neuroprotective in experimental acute ischemic stroke. J Cereb Blood Flow Metab. 2016;36(4):721–30.

38. Fraser JF, Maniskas M, Trout A, Lukins D, Parker L, Stafford WL, et al. Intra-arterial verapamil post-thrombectomy is feasible, safe, and neuroprotective in stroke. J Cereb Blood Flow Metab. 2017;37(11):3531–43.

39. Feng L, Fitzsimmons BF, Young WL, Berman MF, Lin E, Aagaard BDL, et al. Intraarterially administered verapamil as adjunct therapy for cerebral vasospasm: safety and 2-year experience. AJNR Am J Neuroradiol. 2002;23(8):1284–90.

40. Veznedaroglu E. Intraarterial verapamil for neuroprotection in ischemic stroke [Internet]. clinicaltrials.gov; 2022 [cited 2023 Dec 31]. Report No.: NCT03347786. Available from:. https://clinicaltrials.gov/study/NCT03347786

41. Kidwell CS, Jahan R, Gornbein J, Alger JR, Nenov V, Ajani Z, et al. A trial of imaging selection and endovascular treatment for ischemic stroke. N Engl J Med. 2013;368(10):914–23.

42. Ciccone A, Valvassori L, Nichelatti M, Sgoifo A, Ponzio M, Sterzi R, et al. Endovascular treatment for acute ischemic stroke. N Engl J Med. 2013;368(10):904–13.

43. Broderick JP, Palesch YY, Demchuk AM, Yeatts SD, Khatri P, Hill MD, et al. Endovascular therapy after intravenous t-PA versus t-PA alone for stroke. N Engl J Med. 2013;368(10):893–903.
44. Berkhemer OA, Fransen PSS, Beumer D, van den Berg LA, Lingsma HF, Yoo AJ, et al. A randomized trial of intraarterial treatment for acute ischemic stroke. N Engl J Med. 2015;372(1):11–20.
45. Araki H, Uchida K, Yoshimura S, Kurisu K, Shime N, Sakamoto S, et al. Effect of region-wide use of prehospital stroke triage scale on management of patients with acute stroke. J Neurointerv Surg. 2022;14(7):677–82.

Venous Sinus Stenting for Idiopathic Intracranial Hypertension

7

Justin M. Cappuzzo, Steven B. Housley, Muhammad Waqas, Andre Monteiro, Ryan M. Hess, Elad I. Levy, and Adnan H. Siddiqui

---

J. M. Cappuzzo · S. B. Housley · M. Waqas · A. Monteiro · R. M. Hess
Department of Neurosurgery, Jacobs School of Medicine and Biomedical Sciences, University at Buffalo, Buffalo, NY, USA

Department of Neurosurgery, Gates Vascular Institute at Kaleida Health, Buffalo, NY, USA
e-mail: j.cappuzzo@atlanticbrainandspine.com; Bhousley@neuroknox.com; mwaqas@ubns.com; amonteiro@ubns.com; rhess@ubns.com

E. I. Levy · A. H. Siddiqui (✉)
Department of Neurosurgery, Jacobs School of Medicine and Biomedical Sciences, University at Buffalo, Buffalo, NY, USA

Department of Neurosurgery, Gates Vascular Institute at Kaleida Health, Buffalo, NY, USA

Department of Radiology, Jacobs School of Medicine and Biomedical Sciences, University at Buffalo, Buffalo, NY, USA

Canon Stroke and Vascular Research Center, University at Buffalo, Buffalo, NY, USA

Jacobs Institute, Buffalo, NY, USA
e-mail: elevy@ubns.com; asiddiqui@ubns.com

© The Author(s), under exclusive license to Springer Nature Switzerland AG 2025
E. Veznedaroglu (ed.), *Advanced Technologies in Vascular Neurosurgery*, https://doi.org/10.1007/978-3-031-67492-1_7

Abbreviations

ACT	Activated clotting time
AP	Anteroposterior
CBF	Cerebral blood flow
CSF	Cerebrospinal fluid
CT	Computed tomography
CTV	Computed tomography venography
DAPT	Dual antiplatelet therapy
DSV	Digital subtraction venography
F	French
GA	General anesthesia
ICP	Intracranial pressure
IIH	Idiopathic intracranial hypertension
LA	Lateroanterior
LP	Lumbar puncture
MR	Magnetic resonance
MRV	Magnetic resonance venography
ONSF	Optic nerve sheath fenestration
PRU	P2Y12 reaction unit
PTC	Pseudotumor cerebri
SSS	Superior sagittal sinus
TOF	Time-of-flight
VSOO	Venous sinus outflow obstruction

Introduction

Idiopathic intracranial hypertension (IIH), previously known as pseudotumor cerebri (PTC), is a neurological condition in which intracranial pressures (ICPs) are elevated in the absence of an underlying mass lesion or dilated ventricular system and is manifested by progressive headaches, papilledema, vision loss, and occasionally pulsatile tinnitus [1]. The incidence of IIH in the general population is approximately 0.9 cases per 100,000 individuals; however, among women aged 20–44 years who are 20% over their ideal body weight, this incidence rises to approximately

19 per 100,000 individuals [2]. Several etiologies have been hypothesized, such as increased cerebral spinal fluid (CSF) production, inadequate CSF resorption, parenchymal edema, venous outflow obstruction, and increased intracerebral blood volume [3–6]. In patients in whom IIH is refractory to conservative management and medical therapy (including weight loss, acetazolamide, topiramate, or diuretics) or who are at significant risk of impending vision loss [7], interventional treatments are warranted. Optic nerve sheath fenestration has been traditionally used for patients who present predominantly with papilledema or vision loss. Ventriculoperitoneal or lumboperitoneal shunting has been favored for patients presenting with headache as the most prominent symptom [8, 9]. More recently, venous sinus stenting arose as an alternative treatment with promising results in refractory IIH patients with severe stenosis of the venous sinuses [1] (Fig. 7.1).

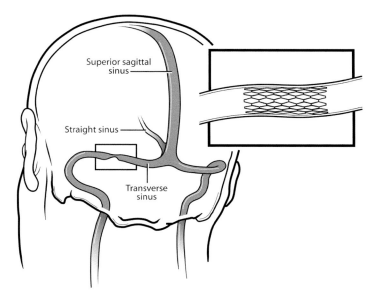

Fig. 7.1 Illustration of severe right mid-transverse sinus stenosis and subsequent stent deployment. (From: Cappuzzo et al. [1])

Although the inciting pathophysiology of IIH remains unclear, venous sinus outflow obstruction (VSOO) has been observed in a large proportion of these patients, with abnormally high-pressure gradients across the stenotic segment. According to Levitt et al., 93% of IIH patients have some degree of venous sinus stenosis [10]. A normal pressure gradient is generally accepted to be <8 mm Hg, and the maximal normal pressure in the superior sagittal sinus (SSS) to be <18 mm Hg [11]. In a systematic review by McDougall et al. in 2018, patients with pressure gradients and venous sinus stenosis showed improvement in their IIH symptoms with venous sinus stenting [12]. Given these findings, it is no surprise that venous sinus stenting has become more favorable than traditional surgical approaches, and clinical trials and studies are ongoing.

In this chapter, the authors briefly discuss the pathophysiology and diagnosis of IIH. They discuss the indications and role of venous sinus stenting for IIH, with an in-depth literature review including present clinical trials. They additionally discuss the technical setup for a diagnostic venogram, lumbar puncture, and venous sinus stenting including nuisances in their technique.

Pathophysiology and Diagnosis of Idiopathic Intracranial Hypertension

Increased CSF Production

Initially, CSF overproduction was postulated to be the main mechanism of IIH; however, contrary to such a theory, CSF hypersecretion is also present in patients with other conditions, such as choroid plexus hyperplasia or choroid plexus papilloma [13]. Additionally, most IIH patients present with normal or reduced ventricular caliber, which suggests that CSF hypersecretion is unlikely to be the pathologic driving force behind this condition [14].

Decreased Reabsorption and Venous Outflow Obstruction

Decreased CSF absorption in arachnoid granulations has also been postulated to be a potential cause of IIH. Obesity, specifically in those with a more central distribution of adipose tissue, increases the intra-abdominal pressure leading to elevated pulmonary and cardiac filling pressures, which in turn decreases venous return to the heart, generating an elevated pressure in the venous system that builds up to the cerebral venous sinuses [15]. Due to elevated pressure, the gradient prevents resorption of CSF into the sinuses through the arachnoid granulations. Furthermore, according to Fargen's unifying theory, the increased ICP can result in collapse of the venous sinus in susceptible segments, thus generating stenosis, which in turn increases even more from the pressure in the dural sinuses due to venous outflow obstruction, in a vicious feedback loop [16]. Therefore, venous hypertension is likely the most reasonable explanation for IIH and why increased ICP is not married to ventricular caliber [17]. This is further validated in studies showing that as SSS pressure elevates, so does CSF pressure secondary to decreased, pressure-dependent absorption of CSF across arachnoid granulations [17–19]. This is the most presently accepted mechanism for the pathophysiology of IIH and will be discussed further later in the chapter.

Increased Intracranial Blood Volume

First proposed by Dandy in 1937, increased intracranial blood volume leading to a shift in the Monro-Kellie doctrine has been thought to contribute to the pathogenesis of IIH [17]. In a positron emission tomography evaluation, Raichle et al. demonstrated that there is little change in cerebral blood flow (CBF) but an increase in cerebral blood volume in these patients [20]. Conversely, in their retrospective studies, Bateman et al. found a 46% increase in CBF, and Bicakci et al. demonstrated IIH patients with both increased and decreased CBF and no difference in cerebral blood volume [21, 22]. Ultimately, this proposed mechanism is still controversial but nonetheless should be further evaluated. The authors of this chapter opine that increases in cerebral blood volume may be secondary to outflow obstructions from increased intra-abdominal and intracardiac pressures and/or venous sinus stenosis.

Diagnosis

The diagnosis of IIH is traditionally based on the modified Dandy criteria (Table 7.1) [23]. A slight adjustment in these criteria was made in 2014 to include patients with a CSF opening pressure of >25 cm H_2O [23, 24]. Initial evaluation in patients with signs and symptoms of IIH consisted of magnetic resonance (MR) imaging to exclude additional pathologies, followed by lumbar puncture (LP). In the past, there were concerns regarding the accuracy of this approach for measuring ICPs; however, Fargen et al. in 2020 reported a series of 104 patients, validating a correlation between the pressures in the lumbar cistern and those in the SSS [11]. Additional imaging, such as MR venography (MRV) or computed tomography (CT) venography, can be used as a preliminary tool for evaluation of the cerebral venous sinuses. "Gold standard" evaluation of venous sinus anatomy and pathology is done with digital subtraction venography (DSV) under conscious sedation. Importantly, conscious sedation is the best method for evaluation when tolerated by the patient, because the performance of venous manometry measurements during DSV has been shown to be significantly altered and potentially nondiagnostic under general anesthesia (GA) [25].

Table 7.1 Diagnosis of idiopathic intracranial hypertension (pseudotumor cerebri)

Modified Dandy criteria

1. Signs and symptoms of increased intracranial pressure (headaches, nausea, vomiting, transient obscurations of vision, papilledema)

2. No localizing neurologic signs otherwise, with the single exception being unilateral or bilateral VI nerve paresis

3. CSF can show increased pressure but no cytologic or chemical abnormalities otherwise

4. Normal to small symmetric ventricles must be demonstrated (originally required ventriculography but now demonstrated by CT)

Diagnostic criteria from 2002

1. If symptoms present, they may only reflect those of generalized intracranial hypertension or papilledema

2. If signs present, they may only reflect those of generalized intracranial hypertension or papilledema

3. Documented elevated intracranial pressure measured in the lateral decubitus position

4. Normal CSF composition

5. No evidence of hydrocephalus, mass, structural, or vascular lesion on MRI or contrast-enhanced CT for typical patients and MRI and MRV for all others

6. No other causes of intracranial hypertension identified

Diagnostic criteria from 2018

1. Required for diagnosis[a]

   A. Papilledema

   B. Normal neurologic examination except for cranial nerve abnormalities

   C. Neuroimaging: normal brain parenchyma without evidence of hydrocephalus, mass, or structural lesion and no abnormal meningeal enhancement on MRI, with and without gadolinium, for typical patients (female and obese), and MRI, with and without gadolinium, and MRV for others; if MRI is unavailable or contraindicated, contrast-enhanced CT may be used

   D. Normal CSF composition

   E. Elevated lumbar puncture opening pressure ($\geq$25 mm H_2O)

(continued)

Table 7.1 (continued)

2. Diagnosis without papilledema
In the absence of papilledema, a diagnosis of pseudotumor cerebri syndrome can be made if B–E above are satisfied, and in addition the patient has a unilateral or bilateral VI nerve palsy
In the absence of papilledema or VI nerve palsy, a diagnosis of pseudotumor cerebri syndrome can be suggested but not made if B–E from the above are satisfied, and, in addition, at least three of the following neuroimaging criteria are satisfied:
(i) Empty sella
(ii) Flattening of the posterior aspect of the globe
(iii) Distention of the perioptic subarachnoid space with or without a tortuous optic nerve
(iv) Transverse venous sinus stenosis

Modified from Friedman and Jacobson [23] and Friedman et al. [24]

Abbreviations: *CSF* cerebrospinal fluid, *CT* computed tomography, *MR* magnetic resonance, *MRI* magnetic resonance imaging, *MRV* magnetic resonance venography

[a]A diagnosis of pseudotumor cerebri syndrome is definite if the patient fulfills criteria A–E. The diagnosis is considered probable if criteria A–D are met, but the measured CSF pressure is lower than specified for a definite diagnosis

Management

The flow diagram in Fig. 7.2 illustrates the general management of patients with IIH and venous sinus stenosis.

Conservative

Weight loss and medical therapy with carbonic anhydrase inhibitors (e.g., acetazolamide) are the first-line options for treatment of IIH. In a randomized controlled trial of 165 patients (IIH Treatment Trial) with mild vision deficit, acetazolamide was shown to improve global visual field loss, papilledema, CSF opening pressure, and vision-related quality of life at 6 months [26]. Topiramate has benefitted these patients due to its mild carbonic anhydrase activity, effective migraine relief, and weight loss side effect [27]. Loop diuretics and corticosteroids have been used in those unable to tolerate acetazolamide or topiramate, but

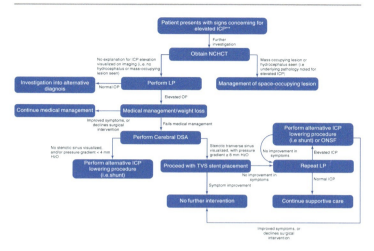

Fig. 7.2 Flow diagram illustrating the general treatment algorithm for patients with IIH and venous sinus stenosis. For those patients presenting with worsening visual symptoms, we are more likely to bypass medical management and proceed directly to DSV if LP OP is elevated. DSV digital subtraction venography, ICP intracranial pressure, LP lumbar puncture, NCHCT noncontrast head computed tomography, ONSF optic nerve sheath fenestration, OP opening pressure, TVS transverse venous stent. (*Source:* Cappuzzo et al. [1]) **For patients presenting with worsening visual symptoms, we are more likely to bypass medical management and proceed directly to digital subtraction angiography if the lumbar puncture opening pressure is elevated

the results are conflicting [7]. Unfortunately, a considerable number of patients—approximately 20%—are refractory to weight loss and medical therapy, or even have worsening of symptoms, requiring more invasive measures to preserve vision and improve quality of life [28].

Surgical Treatment

Optic Nerve Sheath Fenestration (ONSF)

In patients presenting with predominantly papilledema and visual symptoms, ONSF is a reasonable treatment. Several studies have shown its utility in preventing visual decline [29, 30] and providing resolution of papilledema in most patients [31]. The most common surgical approach for ONSF is a transconjunctival medial orbitotomy, which provides good visualization of the optic nerve including anatomical landmarks, a description of which can be found in an article by Mudumbai in 2014 [31]. Alternative approaches include lateral orbitotomy and the upper eyelid approach [32, 33].

Cerebrospinal Fluid Diversion

CSF diversion can be performed through multiple shunting variations, such as ventriculoperitoneal, ventriculopleural, ventriculoatrial, ventriculojugular, and lumboperitoneal shunt placement [9]. This treatment modality is used for patients presenting with both papilledema and headaches, more preferably in cases with headaches as the predominant symptom [9]. Although initial headache relief is achieved along with stability or improvement of papilledema, recurrence rates are high and recurrence is commonly reported. According to a study by Sinclair et al. in 2011, more than 50% of patients require at least one shunt revision, more than 30% require multiple revisions, and headaches (either baseline or low pressure) progressively return over time [34]. Furthermore, shunting can potentially lead to complications such as, but not limited to, infection and hardware failure. Additionally, most patients with IIH have slit-like ventricles, increasing the technical difficulty of shunting procedures.

Venous Sinus Stenting

Background

As previously discussed, the presently most accepted theory for the pathophysiology of IIH is that it is caused by venous hypertension secondary to outflow obstruction, resulting in elevated ICP and its respective clinical manifestations. One of the first observations between venous outflow obstruction (other than venous thrombosis) and IIH symptoms occurred in 1986, when a patient with a cholesteatoma compressing the sigmoid sinus developed IIH-like symptoms that resolved after cyst resection [35]. Just 2 years earlier, another case report had described two patients with posterior sagittal sinus compression resulting in impaired venous drainage and visual loss [36]. More recently, venous outflow obstruction and obstructed CSF absorption are observed to be due to sinus stenosis [37]. Stenosis of the transverse–sigmoid sinuses was first noted in the 1990s in patients presenting with pulsatile tinnitus, and, at that time, stenosis (if present) was thought to be overlooked on noninvasive imaging [38].

Time-of-flight (TOF) MRV became a more frequently used tool in the 1990s, but the imaging quality was poor—one of the transverse sinuses often appeared absent [39]. In the 2000s, different sequences and protocols were implemented to improve the accuracy of the imaging [40–42]. Initially, stenoses were thought to be artifacts of TOF MRV, but improvements in this technology and later correlation with pressure monitoring during DSV determined stenosis to be a real phenomenon in up to 90% of IIH patients [42, 43]. Presently, MRV imaging is touted as the most sensitive noninvasive imaging modality for the detection of transverse sinus stenosis [44].

Stenosis of the venous sinuses can be described as either intrinsic or extrinsic [43]. Intrinsic stenosis refers to an intravascular obstruction (e.g., a large arachnoid granulation) that typically appears as a focal process [45]. Extrinsic stenosis refers to extravascular compression of the venous sinus due to elevated ICP or anatomical variants, resulting in venous outflow obstruction and further increase in ICP and triggering or worsening of IIH symptoms. It typically appears as a long, tapered, and smooth narrowing [45]. King et al. provided some evidence that elevated ICP is a potential cause of venous sinus stenosis when they demonstrated that the removal of 20–25 ml of CSF through C1–2 punctures resulted in return to normal pressure gradients (<8 mm Hg) in most patients in their series [46]. One of their patients continued to have a gradient; however, this was not commented on by the authors [46]. King et al. did note that patients with minocycline-induced IIH did not have gradients, which alludes to the heterogeneity of this disease process [46].

In several studies, the authors have reported that venous sinus stenosis is a consequence and not a primary cause of IIH [47–51]. Other authors have suggested that chronic elevated ICP may result in irreversible sequelae, such as fibrosis and fixed stenosis of the transverse sinus [37, 52, 53]. In even more dramatic cases of chronically elevated ICP, conformational changes in bony anatomy have been observed in the groove occupied by the transverse sinus [54].

Therefore, the existing evidence suggests that IIH is a complex, dynamic, and heterogeneous disease process, without a one-size-fits-all approach. We advise a complete neurosurgical evaluation (discussed later in this chapter) of each patient to ensure that the proper treatment modality is chosen. Stenosis can be attributable to various etiologies other than the aforementioned ones, such as mastoiditis, scalp infection, Behcet's disease, or any mass-occupying lesions, all of which are better managed by addressing the underlying cause [46]. A large proportion of patients with IIH do not have sinus stenosis but still have elevated central pressures with a diffuse pressure gradient that is not amenable to endovascular stenting. These patients benefit from weight loss as the mainstay of treatment. Additionally, some patients that do not have stenosis at the transverse–sigmoid sinus instead have it present within the SSS, with no signs of intrinsic stenosis. Regardless of whether this stenosis is causative or resultant, it is clearly related to the overall disease process [37].

Outcomes

The first case of endovascular stenting for venous sinus stenosis was reported in 2002 by Higgins et al. in a young woman with IIH-related symptoms refractory to medical therapy and only transient improvement after an LP [55]. She had bilateral stenoses of the transverse sinuses and a pressure gradient of 18 mm Hg on the dominant side (right). Stenting was performed with a self-expanding stent (EZ Wallstent, Boston Scientific, Marlborough, Massachusetts) achieving a reduction of the pressure gradient to 3 mm Hg, improvement of headaches on the following day, and resolution of papilledema within the 3-week follow-up period [55]. This report initiated a trend toward the evaluation of IIH patients with refractory symptoms as candidates for stenting.

Within the two decades after the initial report, several other operators and centers reported successful treatment of IIH patients with sinus stenosis using stenting in case series and literature reviews [28, 37, 43, 56–66]. In 2017, the first two prospective trials were published [67, 68]. Dinkin et al. designed their trial to include 13 IIH patients with symptoms that were refractory to or who were intolerant to medical therapy or who presented with acute vision loss and evidence of transverse–sigmoid sinus stenosis with a gradient of 8 mm Hg or higher [67]. If stenosis was present bilaterally, the nondominant side was stented [67]. Patients were kept on aspirin (325 mg) plus clopidogrel (75 mg) daily for 1 month, after which only aspirin (325 mg) was maintained for 6 months [67]. The precise stent (Cordis, Fremont, California) was used, with diameters ranging from 8 to 10 mm and lengths ranging from 30 to 40 mm [67]. Of the patients included in the study, 84.7% had improvement in their headaches, 100% had improvement in pulsatile tinnitus, and 11 patients had improved vision [67].

Concomitantly, Liu et al. reported their prospective clinical trial including ten patients with medically refractory IIH and documented visual changes adjudicated by an ophthalmologist [68]. Stenting was offered to patients who were found to have venous sinus stenosis with elevated ICP ≥26 mm Hg (measured via right frontal ICP monitor) and increased pressure gradient (≥16 mm Hg) in addition to signs and symptoms of IIH [68]. Improvement was seen in nine (90%) of patients over a follow-up period of 15–32 months. Stenosis adjacent to the stent recurred in two (20%) patients, who were all successfully treated with a new stenting procedure [68]. Papilledema improvement was documented in all ten patients on follow-up funduscopic testing [68]. Liu et al. used a Wallstent, similar to the device used by Higgins et al. [55, 68].

Due to its design for carotid stenosis, the Wallstent is a rather rigid stent that was not flexible enough to conform to the anatomy surrounding the transverse–sigmoid region. Eventually, newer stents with better conformability were used for the purpose of venous sinus stenting, such as the Zilver drug-eluting peripheral stent (Cook Medical, Bloomington, Indiana) and the Acculink carotid stent (Abbott, Lake Bluff, Illinois) [1, 8, 11, 69–71]. The most recent review by Leishangthem et al. included 29 studies comprising 410 IIH patients, with an overall high technical success rate (99.5%), low rate of repeat procedure (10%), and a low major complication rate (1.5%) [45]. In a systematic review and meta-analysis of 474 patients with IIH, Nicholson et al. demonstrated an improvement in papilledema in 93.7%, improvement in headache in 79.6%, and resolution of pulsatile tinnitus in 90.3%, with an overall rate of symptom recurrence in 9.8% [72]. In our experience, venous sinus stenting typically produces a rapid improvement in the patient's pressure gradient, and improvement in symptoms can be seen immediately following the procedure in some instances, with most patients noting significant improvement in the days–weeks following the procedure.

Prestenting Evaluation

All patients are seen in our outpatient clinics for a full neurosurgical evaluation including a thorough history and physical examination. Patients with history and symptoms consistent with IIH are referred to an ophthalmologist for a detailed eye examination including fundoscopy, visual fields, and acuity testing. These patients are also referred to the neurology service for medical therapy management in the interim. Noninvasive imaging is obtained; MRV is preferred because of its nonradioactive exposure compared to CT venography (CTV). If any degree of stenosis along the venous sinuses is detected on noninvasive imaging, the patient is scheduled for a biplane fluoroscopy-guided LP and diagnostic DSV, with both performed under conscious sedation. We have found that although an LP can easily be performed at the bedside, performing it under conscious sedation and fluoroscopy is more comfortable for the patient and makes the opening pressure more accurate by avoiding a false elevation. The patient is placed in the lateral decubitus position to ensure that there are no external sources of compression (such as abdominal pressure on the bed) that can falsely elevate the ICP (Fig. 7.3). Similarly, we perform our diagnostic venogram under conscious sedation, as it decreases recovery and intraoperative fluoroscopy time. In our experience, although lower pressure measurements have been

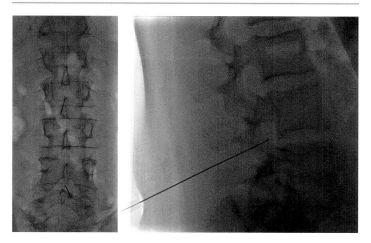

Fig. 7.3 Fluoroscopic-guided lumbar puncture (LP) at the L4–5 level in the anteroposterior (AP) (left) and lateroanterior (LA) (right) planes. The opening pressure in this particular case was noted to be 63 cm H_2O Hg. The key to a successful LP is to use biplane fluoroscopy first in the AP plane to square off the endplates and separate the spinous processes and enter at midline in a perpendicular fashion and advance the needle. Once the advancement of the needle begins, the LA plane can be used to visualize the needle going toward the spinal canal. Once this is visualized and the ligamentum flavum is felt to be breached, the stylet is removed to reveal cerebrospinal fluid. The patient's legs are straightened, and pressure on the abdomen is released to ensure that accurate, relaxed pressure measurements can be obtained

obtained with GA compared to moderate conscious sedation, the gradients do not change, thereby making moderate conscious sedation our sedation of choice.

The diagnostic venogram is traditionally performed via a transfemoral venous approach. The patient's groin is prepared and draped in the usual sterile fashion. Venipuncture is performed using a 20-gauge micropuncture needle on a 10-ml syringe under aspiration at an acute angle, directly medial to where the femoral artery is palpated. Ultrasound guidance may be used to demonstrate the compressible femoral vein medial to the pulsatile femoral artery. Additionally, with the ultrasound, we can ensure that the venotomy site is not high by identifying the bifurcation of the femoral artery and staying just above the bifurcation. This limits the risk for a retroperitoneal hematoma. Once blood is readily aspirated into the syringe, thus confirming placement of the needle within the vein, the syringe is disconnected and a low-flow state is visually confirmed. A microwire is then placed into the needle with fluoroscopic visualization to confirm placement within the common femoral vein toward the inferior vena cava. Modified Seldinger technique is used to place a 6-French (F) sheath with a J-wire. The three-way stopcock attached to the copilot is turned to confirm the intravascular position of the sheath. A common femoral venous injection may be performed to confirm the sheath position as well as ensure that no extravasation has occurred. We then introduce a 6-F, 95-cm Benchmark catheter (Penumbra Inc., Alameda, California) over a Berenstein catheter (Merit Medical Systems, South Jordan, Utah) over a 0.035-inch exchange length Glidewire (Terumo Interventional Systems, Somerset, New Jersey), and the system is advanced upward via the vena cava to the dominant-sided transverse sinus. Preoperative imaging is used to confirm the dominant side and evaluate for any thrombosis or other outflow obstruction. If sinus thrombosis is a concern, a diagnostic cerebral angiogram can be performed prior to the venogram for evaluation.

The Benchmark catheter is advanced toward the internal jugular–sigmoid sinus interface over the Berenstein catheter and 0.035-inch Glidewire. From here, the Berenstein catheter and Glidewire are removed, and a 160-cm 3Max reperfusion catheter (Penumbra Inc.) is introduced over a 215-cm Synchro-Select Support microwire (Stryker Neurovascular, Fremont, California) toward the SSS. We have found that this microwire provides greater support in traversing the 3Max to the SSS if there is a high-grade stenosis. Alternatively, a 0.035-inch Glidewire may be used through the 3Max if it cannot be navigated with the microwire. Once within the anterior SSS, a puff of contrast material is injected via a 10-ml syringe to confirm placement within the SSS and not in a small cortical vein. Once this is confirmed, a full run is performed. We have found that the ideal views for the anteroposterior (AP) are a Towne's view and for the lateroanterior (LA) any view to offset the left and right transverse–sigmoid sinus junctions from each other (Fig. 7.4a). Any evidence of

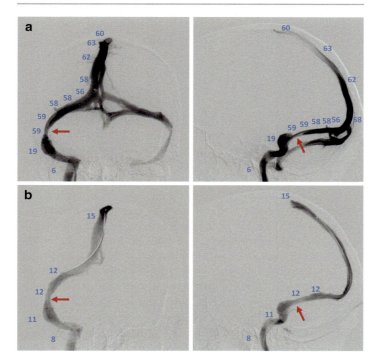

Fig. 7.4 (**a**) Diagnostic cerebral venogram, superior sagittal sinus (SSS) cranial injection in AP (left) and LA (right) planes demonstrating a dominant right transverse sinus with severe stenosis noted at the transverse–sigmoid junction (*arrow in each image*) with a gradient of 50 mm Hg. The pressure measurements at each major anatomical location are listed from superior to inferior, and units are provided in mm Hg: anterior SSS [60], mid-SSS [63], posterior SSS [62], torcula [58], right proximal transverse sinus [56], right mid-transverse sinus [58], right distal transverse sinus [58], right transverse–sigmoid junction [59], right proximal sigmoid sinus [59], right distal sigmoid sinus [19], and right internal jugular bulb [6]. (**b**) Diagnostic cerebral venogram, SSS cranial injection in AP (left) and LA (right) planes demonstrating a dominant right transverse sinus following stent placement using a 9 mm × 60 mm Zilver stent (Cook Medical, Bloomington, Indiana) with improvement seen in the pressure gradient and stenosis (*arrow in each image*). The pressure measurements at each major anatomical location from superior to inferior with units in mm Hg are provided: anterior SSS [15], right transverse sinus [12], right transverse–sigmoid junction [12], right sigmoid sinus [11], and right internal jugular bulb [8]. (**c**) Fluoroscopic X-ray of the skull demonstrating the Zilver stent within the right transverse–sigmoid sinus (left, AP view; right, lateral view)

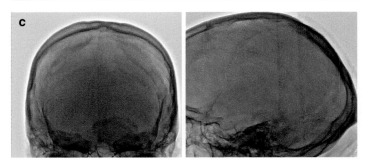

Fig. 7.4 (continued)

sinus stenosis is noted. A pressure monitor is then zeroed and attached to the 3Max catheter, and pressures are taken at the following locations: anterior SSS, mid-SSS, posterior SSS, torcula, proximal transverse sinus, mid-transverse sinus, distal transverse sinus, proximal sigmoid sinus, distal sigmoid sinus, and internal jugular bulb. Additionally, if there is no evidence of a gradient, we note the pressure measurements all the way down toward the superior vena cava. In some instances where there is no focal region of stenosis, there is evidence of central venous hypertension, indicating that the patient typically has an obesity-induced central hypertension and likely would benefit from weight loss.

The pressures of the dominant-sided sinus system are measured; however, if the sinuses are codominant, we typically measure the contralateral pressures as well. If feasible, we cross the torcula to the contralateral transverse sinus with the 3Max catheter and Synchro microwire and measure pressures from the internal jugular bulb back toward the torcula. If bilateral disease exists, the larger (dominant) of the two sides is typically treated.

Indications for Sinus Stenting and Present Trials

Once a patient has:

- Signs and symptoms of IIH.
- Evidence of papilledema.
- Sinus stenosis (usually transverse/sigmoid) in the dominant sinus.
- Focal pressure gradient across the stenosis ≥ 8 mm H_2O.

A gradient of ≥ 8 mm H_2O was first utilized by Dinkin et al. in their initial series of 13 patients and has continued in present-day trials and practice [67, 73]. The Venous Sinus Stenting with the River Stent in IIH trial is an ongoing prospective, multicenter, single-arm, open-label clinical trial using the Serenity River Stent System (Serenity Medical Inc., Ontario, Canada) that started in 2018 and has been a mainstay for setting a present standard for stenting [73]. The criteria for enrollment in this trial are (1) IIH subjects with significant (>50%) stenosis of the transverse–sigmoid sinus junction and (2) moderate to severe visual field loss or severe headaches that have failed to resolve with medical therapy. The investigators note that "in the absence of this trial, subjects would have been offered a surgical treatment of IIH such as sinus stenting with an off-label device, cerebrospinal fluid shunting, or optic nerve sheath fenestration by the treating physician" [73]. Thus far, 39 patients across ten US centers have been enrolled in this study. In our practice, patients without evidence of papilledema are treated with venous sinus stenting for headaches or other clinical findings, such as pulsatile tinnitus, on occasion if they have failed medical therapy.

A relatively new concept is the treatment of IIH with acute visual loss and venous sinus stenosis in the acute setting. Recently, we have begun performing this procedure in the acute setting and have had success with restoration of vision when performed in the days following visual loss [74, 75]. Similar findings were noted by Zehri et al.; however, in their case series of ten patients, the visual loss was within 8 weeks [75]. Venous sinus stenting is likely to continue as a main treatment for this subset of patients.

Technique

Prestenting, the patient is placed on dual antiplatelet therapy (DAPT) with aspirin and either clopidogrel or ticagrelor. P2Y12 levels are obtained to ensure that the patient is therapeutic on either clopidogrel or ticagrelor. If the patient is not therapeutic on clopidogrel, we convert the clopidogrel to ticagrelor. A level of 208 or higher is considered nontherapeutic (at our center); however, we arbitrarily use a P2Y12 reaction unit (PRU) level of 200 as a cutoff.

The patient is brought to the angiographic suite and sedated using moderate conscious sedation. GA may be induced, which will lower the patient's overall venous pressures, and preliminary evidence supports that conscious sedation pressures are more accurate than those under GA [25]. The patient's groin is prepared and draped in the usual sterile fashion. A hemostat is used to identify the lower aspect of the femoral head, which will serve as our general entry site for the venotomy site. Venipuncture is performed using a 20-gauge micropuncture needle on a 10-ml syringe under aspiration at an acute angle, directly medial to where the femoral artery is palpated. Ultrasound guidance may be used to demonstrate the compressible femoral vein medial to the pulsatile femoral artery. Additionally, with the ultrasound, ensuring that the venotomy site is not high can be achieved by identifying the bifurcation of the femoral artery and staying just above the bifurcation. Once blood is readily aspirated into the syringe, thus confirming placement of the needle within the vein, the syringe is disconnected, and a low-flow state is confirmed. A microwire is then placed into the needle with fluoroscopic visualization to confirm placement within the common femoral vein. Modified Seldinger technique is used to place an 8-F sheath. An InQwire guide wire (Merit Medical Systems) is used instead of a standard J-wire for the greater support it provides and to alleviate the need for a 7-F dilator. Turning the stopcock confirms the intravascular position of the sheath. A common femoral venous injection may be performed to confirm position as well as to ensure no extravasation. The patient is then given heparin (50 units/kg bodyweight), and the activated clotting time (ACT) is checked 5 minutes later.

Concomitantly, an 8-F, 95-cm TracStar catheter (Imperative Care, Campbell, California) is introduced over a 5-F, 130-cm Berenstein Select Catheter (Merit Medical Systems) over a 0.035-inch, 260-cm Advantage Glidewire (Terumo Interventional). This wire has a soft tip similar to the traditional 0.035-inch Glidewire while providing extra support for advancing the guide catheter across the level of stenosis in the transverse–sigmoid sinus junction. The system is brought up through the inferior vena cava to the superior vena cava and to the appropriate side of the affected sinus. The TracStar is brought over the Berenstein over the

Glidewire to the internal jugular vein and sigmoid sinus junction. Of note, we do not treat a hypoplastic sinus, and if both sides have stenosis, we treat the dominant sinus. From here, the Berenstein catheter and the Glidewire are removed, and a 115-cm Navien 072 catheter (Medtronic, Dublin, Ireland) is introduced over a 160-cm 3Max over a 300-cm, 0.014-inch Synchro-Select Support wire. The Navien provides extra support to aid the TracStar in advancing past the stenosis (serial dilator). Additionally, the 0.035-inch Advantage Glidewire is able to provide increased support for this purpose as well, and the 3Max has a large enough inner diameter for using this wire (or the 0.014-inch Synchro-Select Support). The 3Max is advanced to the mid-anterior SSS, and a puff of contrast material is injected, confirming that the catheter is not in a cortical vein, followed by an angiographic run that is then used to view the stenosis for stent placement, pressure monitoring, and roadmap purposes. Once this is performed, the TracStar is brought over the region of stenosis (typically located at the transverse–sigmoid sinus). Everything except the TracStar and 300-cm Synchro-Select Support is then removed. If the 0.035-inch Advantage Glidewire was used instead of the Synchro-Select Support, the Glidewire is then removed, and the Synchro-Select Support wire is introduced along with a peripheral Zilver 518 stent. We typically use a Zilver stent that is 8–10 mm in diameter and 60 mm in length. The sinus is a triangular type of structure; therefore, a measurement is not required to fit the largest dimension of the stent, and often a slightly smaller diameter stent will be appropriate. An exchange length wire is utilized to bring the 3Max catheter back at a later time point for post-stent placement angiographic runs. The Zilver 518 fits a 0.014-in wire system; however, the Zilver PTX is able to utilize a 0.035-inch wire system, which is a good alternative, and it can be beneficial to have the system over a thicker wire for support. Regardless of stent choice, the stent is brought up to the tip of the TracStar guide catheter, and then the TracStar is "unsheathed" back proximal to the stenosis to expose the stent. The stent is then deployed appropriately across the stenosis. The exchange length wire is left in place to remove the stent applicator and exchange length wire in the 3Max catheter for both a run and pressure monitoring. A normal finding is no further evidence of gradient (Fig. 7.4b). Typically, a fluoroscopic X-ray is taken to document in situ stent placement (Fig. 7.4c).

These procedures can be performed under either conscious sedation or GA, with the latter being more time intensive. Both methods will demonstrate resolution of the pressure gradient; however, the overall pressure reading will typically be lower in a GA case due to tight control on respiratory status and, subsequently, ICP. The sheath is sewn in place, and serial partial thromboplastin time levels are obtained every 2 hours until no longer therapeutic. Once this is the case, the sheath is removed, and manual pressure is held at the femoral access site for 15–20 minutes or a vascular clamp is placed. The patient is then admitted to a medical–surgical floor, is discharged the next day, and remains on DAPT for 6 months, followed by aspirin for life. No immediate post-stenting imaging is necessary. A follow-up DSV is performed at the 6-month and 1-year marks.

We typically use self-expanding Zilver stents or the Serenity River stent (if part of that trial) in lieu of a balloon-mounted stent. This agrees with the practice that is reported in the literature. We had a single case that required balloon angioplasty before stent placement. We utilized a Pinnacle Destination sheath (Terumo) parked in the mid-internal jugular vein, a TracStar guide, an NC Emerge dilatation catheter (Boston Scientific), and noncompliant EverCross balloons (Medtronic) over a 300-cm Synchro-Select Support to cross the stenosis. In this particular instance, a compliant Scepter C balloon (MicroVention, Aliso Viejo, California) was used initially; however, treating the stenosis required the noncompliant balloon. After the angioplasty was performed, we were able to successfully deploy the Zilver stent across the stenosis.

Complications and Treatment Failure

Venous sinus stenting is an overall technically successful procedure with a relatively low complication profile [45]. However, as this technique becomes more prevalent as a standard treatment for IIH with venous sinus stenosis, awareness of the major complications associated with the procedure is important. An overall rate of major complications of 1–7% has been reported, with most authors reporting a rate under 2% [6, 45, 66, 72, 76, 77]. Major complications reported in the literature include mainly in-stent thrombosis, access site complications, and intracranial hemorrhage [77]. Townsend et al. reviewed the major and minor complications in their case series of 811 venous sinus stenting procedures and 1466 diagnostic venograms and reported cases of in-stent thrombosis and intracranial hemorrhage [77]. The majority of intracranial hemorrhage were secondary to microsystem perforation, whereas in-stent thrombosis could be secondary to non-clopidogrel responder status or non-heparin responder status [77, 78]. Typically, PRU and ACT levels are obtained for each of our cases.

Recurrent disease adjacent to the stent is seen occasionally; however, Ahmed et al. demonstrated that placement of an additional stent in the adjacent segment resolved these symptoms with a rate of 11.5% for adjacent stenosis in their series [43]. The largest series looking at this phenomenon is by Fargen who reviewed pressure gradients before and after stenting and noticed a pattern for the likely location and frequency of adjacent stenosis [16].

The downside of venous sinus stenting is that the patient is on DAPT, making other interventions, such as bariatric surgery, CSF diversion, or OSNF, higher risk or not possible. Nevertheless, it is rare to perform these procedures in the acute setting, and most patients have discontinued the second antiplatelet agent by the time another surgical intervention would be undertaken. The main side effect profile with DAPT has been reported with nuisance bleeding present in 27% of patients [79].

Summary

Idiopathic intracranial hypertension is a neurological condition characterized by elevated ICPs in the absence of an underlying mass lesion or dilated ventricular system and manifested by progressive headaches, papilledema, vision loss, and occasionally pulsatile tinnitus. Although initially treated with weight loss, carbonic anhydrase inhibitors, and CSF diversion, venous sinus stenting has become a more prevalent treatment when patients are found to have venous sinus stenosis with a severe pressure gradient.

Venous sinus stenting has a high overall technical proficiency rate with a low rate of complications and need for retreatment. Additionally, acute treatment of IIH and venous sinus stenosis with venous sinus stenting in the setting of acute visual loss has shown promising results and may become a front-line therapy in the future. Clinical trials, such as the River stent trial, are presently underway.

Acknowledgments We thank Paul H Dressel BFA for preparation of the figures, Carrie Owens MSILS for formatting the references, and Debra J Zimmer for editorial support.

Disclosure of Relationships/Potential Conflicts of Interest *JMC*—Consulting fees: Cerenovus, J&J Medical Device Companies; Integra LifeSciences, Corp.; MIVI Neuroscience, Inc.; Penumbra, Inc.; Stryker Neurovascular, Corp.; support for attending meetings and/or travel: Stryker, Penumbra.
SBH, MW, AM—None.
RMH—Consulting fees: IRRAS USA, Inc.
EIL—Shareholder/ownership Interest: NeXtGen Biologics, RAPID Medical, Claret Medical, Cognition Medical, Imperative Care, Rebound Therapeutics, StimMed, Three Rivers Medical; Patent: Bone Scalpel; Honorarium for Training & Lectures: Medtronic, Penumbra, MicroVention, Integra, Consultant: Clarion, GLG Consulting, Guidepoint Global, Imperative Care, Medtronic, StimMed, Misionix, Mosaic; Chief Medical Officer: Haniva Technology; National PI: Medtronic—Steering Committees for SWIFT Prime and SWIFT Direct Trials; Site PI Study: MicroVention (CONFIDENCE Study) Medtronic (STRATIS Study-Sub 1); Advisory Board: Stryker (AIS Clinical Advisory Board), NeXtGen Biologics, MEDX, Cognition Medical; Endostream Medical, IRRAS AB (Consultant/Advisory Board, Medical Legal Review: renders medical/legal opinions as an expert witness; Leadership or fiduciary roles in other board society, committee, or advocacy group, paid and unpaid: CNS, ABNS, UBNS.
AHS—Consulting fees: Amnis Therapeutics, Apellis Pharmaceuticals, Inc., Boston Scientific, Canon Medical Systems USA, Inc., Cardinal Health 200, LLC, Cerebrotech Medical Systems, Inc., Cerenovus, Cerevatech Medical, Inc., Cordis, Corindus, Inc., Endostream Medical, Ltd., Imperative Care, InspireMD, Ltd., Integra, IRRAS AB, Medtronic, MicroVention, Minnetronix Neuro, Inc., Peijia Medical, Penumbra, Q'Apel Medical, Inc., Rapid Medical, Serenity Medical, Inc., Silk Road Medical, StimMed, LLC, Stryker Neurovascular, Three Rivers Medical, Inc., VasSol, Viz.ai, Inc. Leadership or fiduciary role in other board, society, committee, or advocacy group:

Secretary—Board of the Society of NeuroInterventional Surgery 2020–2021, Chair—Cerebrovascular Section of the AANS/CNS 2020–2021. Stock or stock options: Adona Medical, Inc., Amnis Therapeutics, Bend, IT Technologies, Ltd., BlinkTBI, Inc., Cerebrotech Medical Systems, Inc., Cerevatech Medical, Inc., Cognition Medical, CVAID Ltd., E8, Inc., Endostream Medical, Ltd., Galaxy Therapeutics, Inc., Imperative; Care, Inc., InspireMD, Ltd., Instylla, Inc., International Medical Distribution Partners, Launch NY, Inc.; Neurolutions, Inc., NeuroRadial Technologies, Inc., NeuroTechnology Investors, Neurovascular Diagnostics, Inc., Peijia; Medical, PerFlow Medical, Ltd., Q'Apel Medical, Inc., QAS.ai, Inc., Radical Catheter Technologies, Inc., Rebound Therapeutics Corp. (purchased 2019 by Integra LifeSciences, Corp.), Rist Neurovascular, Inc. (purchased 2020 by Medtronic), Sense Diagnostics, Inc., Serenity Medical, Inc., Silk Road Medical, Sim & Cure, SongBird Therapy, Spinnaker Medical, Inc., StimMed, LLC, Synchron, Inc., Three Rivers Medical, Inc., Truvic Medical, Inc., Tulavi Therapeutics, Inc., Vastrax, LLC, VICIS, Inc., Viseon, Inc. Other financial or nonfinancial interests: National PI/Steering Committees: Cerenovus EXCELLENT and ARISE II Trial; Medtronic SWIFT PRIME, VANTAGE, EMBOLISE, and SWIFT DIRECT Trials; MicroVention FRED Trial & CONFIDENCE Study; MUSC POSITIVE Trial; Penumbra 3D Separator Trial, COMPASS Trial, INVEST Trial, MIVI neuroscience EVAQ Trial; Rapid Medical SUCCESS Trial; InspireMD C-GUARDIANS IDE Pivotal Trial.

References

1. Cappuzzo JM, Hess RM, Morrison JF, Davies JM, Snyder KV, Levy EI, et al. Transverse venous stenting for the treatment of idiopathic intracranial hypertension, or pseudotumor cerebri. Neurosurg Focus. 2018;45(1):E11.
2. Degnan AJ, Levy LM. Pseudotumor cerebri: brief review of clinical syndrome and imaging findings. AJNR Am J Neuroradiol. 2011;32(11):1986–93.
3. Iencean SM. Simultaneous hypersecretion of CSF and of brain interstitial fluid causes idiopathic intracranial hypertension. Med Hypotheses. 2003;61(5–6):529–32.
4. Johnston I. Reduced C.S.F. absorption syndrome. Reappraisal of benign intracranial hypertension and related conditions. Lancet. 1973;2(7826):418–21.
5. Malm J, Kristensen B, Markgren P, Ekstedt J. CSF hydrodynamics in idiopathic intracranial hypertension: a long-term study. Neurology. 1992;42(4):851–8.

6. Markey KA, Mollan SP, Jensen RH, Sinclair AJ. Understanding idiopathic intracranial hypertension: mechanisms, management, and future directions. Lancet Neurol. 2016;15(1):78–91.

7. Matthews YY. Drugs used in childhood idiopathic or benign intracranial hypertension. Arch Dis Child Educ Pract Ed. 2008;93(1):19–25.

8. McCallum AP, Ding D. Venous sinus stenting for idiopathic intracranial hypertension. In: Mascitelli JR, Binning MJ, editors. Introduction to vascular neurosurgery. Cham: Springer International Publishing; 2022. p. 473–89.

9. Wall M. Idiopathic intracranial hypertension (Pseudotumor cerebri). Curr Neurol Neurosci Rep. 2008;8(2):87–93.

10. Levitt MR, Hlubek RJ, Moon K, Kalani MY, Nakaji P, Smith KA, et al. Incidence and predictors of dural venous sinus pressure gradient in idiopathic intracranial hypertension and non-idiopathic intracranial hypertension headache patients: results from 164 cerebral venograms. J Neurosurg. 2017;126(2):347–53.

11. Fargen KM, Garner RM, Kittel C, Wolfe SQ. A descriptive study of venous sinus pressures and gradients in patients with idiopathic intracranial hypertension. J Neurointerv Surg. 2020;12(3):320–5.

12. McDougall CM, Ban VS, Beecher J, Pride L, Welch BG. Fifty shades of gradients: does the pressure gradient in venous sinus stenting for idiopathic intracranial hypertension matter? A systematic review. J Neurosurg. 2018;130(3):999–1005.

13. Mohanty S, Rout SS, Sarangi GS, Devi K. Choroid plexus papilloma arising from the temporal horn With a bilateral hypersecretory hydrocephalus: a case report and review of literature. World J Oncol. 2016;7(2–3):51–6.

14. Baykan B, Ekizoglu E, Altiokka UG. An update on the pathophysiology of idiopathic intracranial hypertension alias pseudotumor cerebri. Agri. 2015;27(2):63–72.

15. Subramaniam S, Fletcher WA. Obesity and weight loss in idiopathic intracranial hypertension: a narrative review. J Neuroophthalmol. 2017;37(2):197–205.

16. Fargen KM. A unifying theory explaining venous sinus stenosis and recurrent stenosis following venous sinus stenting in patients with idiopathic intracranial hypertension. J Neurointerv Surg. 2021;13(7):587–92.

17. Spennato P, Ruggiero C, Parlato RS, Buonocore MC, Varone A, Cianciulli E, et al. Pseudotumor cerebri. Childs Nerv Syst. 2011;27(2):215–35.

18. Grzybowski DM, Holman DW, Katz SE, Lubow M. In vitro model of cerebrospinal fluid outflow through human arachnoid granulations. Invest Ophthalmol Vis Sci. 2006;47(8):3664–72.

19. Lalou AD, Czosnyka M, Czosnyka ZH, Krishnakumar D, Pickard JD, Higgins NJ. Coupling of CSF and sagittal sinus pressure in adult patients with pseudotumour cerebri. Acta Neurochir. 2020;162(5):1001–9.

20. Raichle ME, Grubb RL Jr, Phelps ME, Gado MH, Caronna JJ. Cerebral hemodynamics and metabolism in pseudotumor cerebri. Ann Neurol. 1978;4(2):104–11.
21. Bicakci K, Bicakci S, Aksungur E. Perfusion and diffusion magnetic resonance imaging in idiopathic intracranial hypertension. Acta Neurol Scand. 2006;114(3):193–7.
22. Bateman GA. Vascular hydraulics associated with idiopathic and secondary intracranial hypertension. AJNR Am J Neuroradiol. 2002;23(7):1180–6.
23. Friedman DI, Jacobson DM. Diagnostic criteria for idiopathic intracranial hypertension. Neurology. 2002;59(10):1492–5.
24. Friedman DI, Liu GT, Digre KB. Revised diagnostic criteria for the pseudotumor cerebri syndrome in adults and children. Neurology. 2013;81(13):1159–65.
25. Raper DMS, Buell TJ, Chen CJ, Ding D, Starke RM, Liu KC. Intracranial venous pressures under conscious sedation and general anesthesia. J Neurointerv Surg. 2017;9(10):986–9.
26. Nordic Idiopathic Intracranial Hypertension Study Group Writing Committee, Wall M, McDermott MP, Kieburtz KD, Corbett JJ, Feldon SE, et al. Effect of acetazolamide on visual function in patients with idiopathic intracranial hypertension and mild visual loss: the idiopathic intracranial hypertension treatment trial. JAMA. 2014;311(16):1641–51.
27. Celebisoy N, Gokcay F, Sirin H, Akyurekli O. Treatment of idiopathic intracranial hypertension: topiramate vs acetazolamide, an open-label study. Acta Neurol Scand. 2007;116(5):322–7.
28. Arac A, Lee M, Steinberg GK, Marcellus M, Marks MP. Efficacy of endovascular stenting in dural venous sinus stenosis for the treatment of idiopathic intracranial hypertension. Neurosurg Focus. 2009;27(5):E14.
29. Chandrasekaran S, McCluskey P, Minassian D, Assaad N. Visual outcomes for optic nerve sheath fenestration in pseudotumour cerebri and related conditions. Clin Exp Ophthalmol. 2006;34(7):661–5.
30. Banta JT, Farris BK. Pseudotumor cerebri and optic nerve sheath decompression. Ophthalmology. 2000;107(10):1907–12.
31. Mudumbai RC. Optic nerve sheath fenestration: indications, techniques, mechanisms and, results. Int Ophthalmol Clin. 2014;54(1):43–9.
32. Pelton RW, Patel BC. Superomedial lid crease approach to the medial intraconal space: a new technique for access to the optic nerve and central space. Ophthal Plast Reconstr Surg. 2001;17(4):241–53.
33. David TT, Nerad JA, Anderson RL, Corbett JJ. Optic nerve sheath fenestration in pseudotumor cerebri: a lateral orbitotomy approach. Arch Opthalmol. 1988;106(10):1458–62.
34. Sinclair AJ, Kuruvath S, Sen D, Nightingale PG, Burdon MA, Flint G. Is cerebrospinal fluid shunting in idiopathic intracranial hypertension worthwhile? A 10-year review. Cephalalgia. 2011;31(16):1627–33.

35. Powers JM, Schnur JA, Baldree ME. Pseudotumor cerebri due to partial obstruction of the sigmoid sinus by a cholesteatoma. Arch Neurol. 1986;43(5):519–21.
36. Repka MX, Miller NR. Papilledema and dural sinus obstruction. J Clin Neuroophthalmol. 1984;4(4):247–50.
37. Kanagalingam S, Subramanian PS. Cerebral venous sinus stenting for pseudotumor cerebri: a review. Saudi J Ophthalmol. 2015;29(1):3–8.
38. Russell EJ, De Michaelis BJ, Wiet R, Meyer J. Objective pulse-synchronous "essential" tinnitus due to narrowing of the transverse dural venous sinus. Int Tinnitus J. 1995;1(2):127–37.
39. Carriero A, Magarelli N, Samuele F, Palumbo L, Bocola V, Iezzi A. The torcular Herophili: the diagnostic pitfalls in TOF 3D magnetic resonance angiography. Radiol Med. 1994;87(4):441–6.
40. Fera F, Bono F, Messina D, Gallo O, Lanza PL, Auteri W, et al. Comparison of different MR venography techniques for detecting transverse sinus stenosis in idiopathic intracranial hypertension. J Neurol. 2005;252(9):1021–5.
41. Ayanzen RH, Bird CR, Keller PJ, McCully FJ, Theobald MR, Heiserman JE. Cerebral MR venography: normal anatomy and potential diagnostic pitfalls. AJNR Am J Neuroradiol. 2000;21(1):74–8.
42. Farb RI, Vanek I, Scott JN, Mikulis DJ, Willinsky RA, Tomlinson G, et al. Idiopathic intracranial hypertension: the prevalence and morphology of sinovenous stenosis. Neurology. 2003;60(9):1418–24.
43. Ahmed RM, Wilkinson M, Parker GD, Thurtell MJ, Macdonald J, McCluskey PJ, et al. Transverse sinus stenting for idiopathic intracranial hypertension: a review of 52 patients and of model predictions. AJNR Am J Neuroradiol. 2011;32(8):1408–14.
44. Morris PP, Black DF, Port J, Campeau N. Transverse sinus stenosis is the most sensitive MR imaging correlate of idiopathic intracranial hypertension. AJNR Am J Neuroradiol. 2017;38(3):471–7.
45. Leishangthem L, SirDeshpande P, Dua D, Satti SR. Dural venous sinus stenting for idiopathic intracranial hypertension: an updated review. J Neuroradiol. 2019;46(2):148–54.
46. King JO, Mitchell PJ, Thomson KR, Tress BM. Manometry combined with cervical puncture in idiopathic intracranial hypertension. Neurology. 2002;58(1):26–30.
47. Baryshnik DB, Farb RI. Changes in the appearance of venous sinuses after treatment of disordered intracranial pressure. Neurology. 2004;62(8):1445–6.
48. Horev A, Hallevy H, Plakht Y, Shorer Z, Wirguin I, Shelef I. Changes in cerebral venous sinuses diameter after lumbar puncture in idiopathic intracranial hypertension: a prospective MRI study. J Neuroimaging. 2013;23(3):375–8.
49. Lee SW, Gates P, Morris P, Whan A, Riddington L. Idiopathic intracranial hypertension; immediate resolution of venous sinus "obstruction" after

reducing cerebrospinal fluid pressure to<10cmH(2)O. J Clin Neurosci. 2009;16(12):1690–2.

50. Stienen A, Weinzierl M, Ludolph A, Tibussek D, Hausler M. Obstruction of cerebral venous sinus secondary to idiopathic intracranial hypertension. Eur J Neurol. 2008;15(12):1416–8.

51. Buell TJ, Raper DMS, Pomeraniec IJ, Ding D, Chen CJ, Taylor DG, et al. Transient resolution of venous sinus stenosis after high-volume lumbar puncture in a patient with idiopathic intracranial hypertension. J Neurosurg. 2018;129(1):153–6.

52. De Simone R, Ranieri A, Bonavita V. Advancement in idiopathic intracranial hypertension pathogenesis: focus on sinus venous stenosis. Neurol Sci. 2010;31(Suppl 1):S33–9.

53. Biousse V, Bruce BB, Newman NJ. Update on the pathophysiology and management of idiopathic intracranial hypertension. J Neurol Neurosurg Psychiatry. 2012;83(5):488–94.

54. Connor SE, Siddiqui MA, Stewart VR, O'Flynn EA. The relationship of transverse sinus stenosis to bony groove dimensions provides an insight into the aetiology of idiopathic intracranial hypertension. Neuroradiology. 2008;50(12):999–1004.

55. Higgins JN, Owler BK, Cousins C, Pickard JD. Venous sinus stenting for refractory benign intracranial hypertension. Lancet. 2002;359(9302):228–30.

56. Higgins JN, Cousins C, Owler BK, Sarkies N, Pickard JD. Idiopathic intracranial hypertension: 12 cases treated by venous sinus stenting. J Neurol Neurosurg Psychiatry. 2003;74(12):1662–6.

57. Ogungbo B, Roy D, Gholkar A, Mendelow AD. Endovascular stenting of the transverse sinus in a patient presenting with benign intracranial hypertension. Br J Neurosurg. 2003;17(6):565–8.

58. Owler BK, Parker G, Halmagyi GM, Dunne VG, Grinnell V, McDowell D, et al. Pseudotumor cerebri syndrome: venous sinus obstruction and its treatment with stent placement. J Neurosurg. 2003;98(5):1045–55.

59. Rajpal S, Niemann DB, Turk AS. Transverse venous sinus stent placement as treatment for benign intracranial hypertension in a young male: case report and review of the literature. J Neurosurg. 2005;102(3 Suppl):342–6.

60. Donnet A, Metellus P, Levrier O, Mekkaoui C, Fuentes S, Dufour H, et al. Endovascular treatment of idiopathic intracranial hypertension: clinical and radiologic outcome of 10 consecutive patients. Neurology. 2008;70(8):641–7.

61. Paquet C, Poupardin M, Boissonnot M, Neau JP, Drouineau J. Efficacy of unilateral stenting in idiopathic intracranial hypertension with bilateral venous sinus stenosis: a case report. Eur Neurol. 2008;60(1):47–8.

62. Puffer RC, Mustafa W, Lanzino G. Venous sinus stenting for idiopathic intracranial hypertension: a review of the literature. J Neurointerv Surg. 2013;5(5):483–6.

63. Teleb MS, Cziep ME, Lazzaro MA, Gheith A, Asif K, Remler B, et al. Idiopathic intracranial hypertension. A systematic analysis of transverse sinus stenting. Interv Neurol. 2013;2(3):132–43.

64. Elder BD, Goodwin CR, Kosztowski TA, Radvany MG, Gailloud P, Moghekar A, et al. Venous sinus stenting is a valuable treatment for fulminant idiopathic intracranial hypertension. J Clin Neurosci. 2015;22(4):685–9.

65. Satti SR, Leishangthem L, Chaudry MI. Meta-analysis of CSF diversion procedures and dural venous sinus stenting in the setting of medically refractory idiopathic intracranial hypertension. AJNR Am J Neuroradiol. 2015;36(10):1899–904.

66. Starke RM, Wang T, Ding D, Durst CR, Crowley RW, Chalouhi N, et al. Endovascular treatment of venous sinus stenosis in idiopathic intracranial hypertension: complications, neurological outcomes, and radiographic results. ScientificWorldJournal. 2015;2015:140408.

67. Dinkin MJ, Patsalides A. Venous sinus stenting in idiopathic intracranial hypertension: results of a prospective trial. J Neuroophthalmol. 2017;37(2):113–21.

68. Liu KC, Starke RM, Durst CR, Wang TR, Ding D, Crowley RW, et al. Venous sinus stenting for reduction of intracranial pressure in IIH: a prospective pilot study. J Neurosurg. 2017;127(5):1126–33.

69. El Mekabaty A, Pearl MS, Moghekar A, Gailloud P. Mid-term assessment of transverse sinus stent patency in 104 patients treated for intracranial hypertension secondary to dural sinus stenosis. J Neurointerv Surg. 2021;13(2):182–6.

70. Lee KE, Zehri A, Soldozy S, Syed H, Catapano JS, Maurer R, et al. Dural venous sinus stenting for treatment of pediatric idiopathic intracranial hypertension. J Neurointerv Surg. 2021;13(5):465–70.

71. Townsend RK, Fargen KM. Intracranial venous hypertension and venous sinus stenting in the modern management of idiopathic intracranial hypertension. Life (Basel). 2021;11(6)

72. Nicholson P, Brinjikji W, Radovanovic I, Hilditch CA, Tsang ACO, Krings T, et al. Venous sinus stenting for idiopathic intracranial hypertension: a systematic review and meta-analysis. J Neurointerv Surg. 2019;11(4):380–5.

73. Venous Sinus Stenting With the River Stent in IIH [Clinical Trial]. 2022 [updated 01/12/2022]. Available from: https://clinicaltrials.gov/ct2/show/NCT03556085#moreinfo.

74. Monteiro AFA, Cappuzzo JM, Waqas M, Levy EI, Siddiqui AH. Venous sinus stenting for the treatment of acute blindness in a patient with idiopathic intracranial hypertension. Interv Neuroradiol. 2022; Interv Neuroradiol 2023;29(5):605–8. https://doi.org/10.1177/15910199221095973. Epub 2022 Apr 26.

75. Zehri AH, Lee KE, Kartchner J, Arnel M, Martin T, Wolfe SQ, et al. Efficacy of dural venous sinus stenting in treating idiopathic intracranial hypertension with acute vision loss. Neuroradiol J. 2022;35(1):86–93.

76. Giridharan N, Patel SK, Ojugbeli A, Nouri A, Shirani P, Grossman AW, et al. Understanding the complex pathophysiology of idiopathic intracranial hypertension and the evolving role of venous sinus stenting: a comprehensive review of the literature. Neurosurg Focus. 2018;45(1):E10.

77. Townsend RK, Jost A, Amans MR, Hui F, Bender MT, Satti SR, et al. Major complications of dural venous sinus stenting for idiopathic intracranial hypertension: case series and management considerations. J Neurointerv Surg. 2022;14(1): neurintsurg-2021-017361. https://doi.org/10.1136/neurintsurg-2021-017361. Epub 2021 Apr 28.

78. Lavoie P, Audet ME, Gariepy JL, Savard M, Verreault S, Gourdeau A, et al. Severe cerebellar hemorrhage following transverse sinus stenting for idiopathic intracranial hypertension. Interv Neuroradiol. 2018;24(1):100–5.

79. Pressman E, De la Garza CA, Chin F, Fishbein J, Waqas M, Siddiqui A, et al. Nuisance bleeding complications in patients with cerebral aneurysm treated with pipeline embolization device. J Neurointerv Surg. 2021;13(3):247–50.

Robotic-Assisted Endovascular Intervention

8

Marcus Wong and Gavin Britz

Introduction

The growth of robotics in neurosurgery has made its greatest impact in functional and spine surgery. The introduction of robotic assistance in the fields of interventional cardiology and vascular surgery has paved the way for neurovascular robotics. Robotic assistance holds the promise of increased navigation and device precision, lower radiation exposure for the patient and primary interventionalist, and future remote capabilities that will increase health service access to patients around the country. In this chapter, we discuss the foundational work of the neurovascular robot, its practical workflow and advantages, its future potential, and present limitations.

History

The first published instance of robotic-assisted vascular intervention was performed in 2011 by Granada et al. who reported on eight patients who underwent percutaneous coronary intervention

M. Wong · G. Britz (✉)
Department of Neurosurgery, Houston Methodist Neurological Institute, Houston, TX, USA
e-mail: gbritz@Houstonmethodist.org

© The Author(s), under exclusive license to Springer Nature Switzerland AG 2025
E. Veznedaroglu (ed.), *Advanced Technologies in Vascular Neurosurgery*, https://doi.org/10.1007/978-3-031-67492-1_8

135

[1]. In that series, there was a 97.9% success rate and a 97% decrease in radiation exposure. These results were followed by the Percutaneous Robotically Enhanced Coronary Intervention (PRECISE) study and Complex Robotically Assisted Percutaneous Coronary Intervention (CORA-PCI) study. They found a 97.5% success rate and 95% decrease in radiation exposure in 164 patients requiring a single coronary stent and 91.7% technical and 99.1% clinical success rate in 334 PCIs performed by a single operator, respectively [2, 3]. The success of these studies opened the door for peripheral vascular work in the Robotic-Assisted Peripheral Interventional (RAPID) trial for critical limb ischemia and claudication of the femoropopliteal arteries. Here, the authors demonstrated 100% technical success rate and shorter fluoroscopy times in robotic-assisted interventions [4]. The robotic system used in this trial was the CorPath 200 by Corindus, and its success secured FDA approval for its use in peripheral vascular disease and PCI.

Robotic-Assisted Endovascular Work

On the heels of this success in the cardiac and vascular fields, robotic assistance set its sights on neurointervention. There were some gaps to bridge, however. In contrast to the aforementioned fields, neurovascular intervention often requires a triaxial system with need for microvascular support. Critically, the intracranial space has very little margin for error, and small unintended movements of the microcatheter can lead to disastrous results. To address these concerns, Britz et al. tested and suggested hardware and software modifications for the updated system, the CorPath GRX. That group first successfully used the robot in vitro in an aneurysm flow model to navigate a microcatheter, deploy and bare metal stent, and deliver two coils (Fig. 8.1) [5]. These interventions were made possible by the addition of active device fixation. This allows microcatheter movement without changing the position of the guidewire, thereby reducing the risk of unintentional wire movement and reducing the risk of vessel perforation. Further, the same group performed robotic navigation in extracranial carotid branches in a porcine model. These vessels are

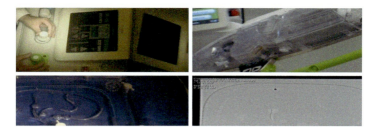

Fig. 8.1 Operational set up demonstrating remote control of endovascular robot to navigate and coil a flow model

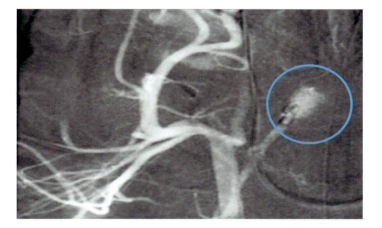

Fig. 8.2 Robotic navigation and coiling of porcine *rete mirabile (blue)*

bioequivalent in size to intracranial human arteries. These were possible with the addition of a second Y adaptor to accommodate and enable the use of the microcatheter [5]. These device modifications and testing led to the CorPath GRX's approval for the European Conformity (CE) mark for neurovascular work. There is still no FDA approval at this time.

The Britz group continued its work, demonstrating the feasibility of robotic-assisted AVM embolization via four *rete mirabile* embolizations in a swine model (Fig. 8.2) [6]. Most recently, Britz and Lumsden also performed a proof-of-concept study to perform a carotid artery stent and mechanical thrombectomy in a fresh-frozen cadaver through a transcarotid artery approach utilizing the TCAR system [7]. Carotid artery stenting has also previously been performed in the discontinued Magellan robotic system in 13 patients with 100% technical success and no neurologic adverse effects postoperatively [8].

The first in-human intracranial work was performed in Canada in 2020 to treat a basilar aneurysm via stent-assisted coiling [9]. Since then, six patients have undergone robotic-assisted embolization by the same group. Four of these were neck-bridging stents, and two flow-diverting stents. These were performed with 100% technical success without morbidity or mortality. At 1-year follow-up, four of the aneurysms were completely occluded, while two had a residual neck [10]. Britz et al. reported the first in-human extracranial embolization series in six patients without any complication [11]. In 2022, Tateshima et al. reported on the first case of robotic-assisted spinal angiography [11]. Here, the authors manually performed the balloon angioplasty and deployment of stents for carotid interventions. The CorPath GRX was able to navigate the balloon and stent to the desired location, but there was no robotic mechanism for their final deployment. Sajja et al. described their experience with ten carotid artery stenting procedures. The same group later compared the robotic-assisted transradial carotid stent to the manual transradial approach and found that the robotic group took significantly longer time and required one conversion to transfemoral. There otherwise was 100% technical success rate without morbidity [12, 13].

CorPath GRX System

The CorPath GRX is the last version of the Corindus endovascular system. It includes an interventional cockpit, which is comprised of a radiation shield, console panel, and monitors, as well as the bedside unit that can be mounted on the operating table. The console panel has a touchscreen, a turbo button for faster tool movement, and three joysticks, which are used to control the guide catheter, guidewire, and interventional devices such as balloons or stents. The addition of the third joystick, a bedside touchscreen, and active guide control, which enables the ability to advance, retract, and rotate the guide catheter, separates the GRX from the previous CorPath 200 version. The monitors display essential angio suite views, such as the live fluoroscopy images, vital signs, and saved angiographic images. The bedside unit handles a flexible robotic arm that is guided to an optimal position for the access site. Importantly, there is a single-use cassette that holds the guiding catheter, guidewire, and a stent or balloon catheter. The cassette also includes a support track that holds the guiding catheter in place and prevents it from bending when the catheter is advanced or retracted or during device exchanges (Fig. 8.3).

In its present iteration, the system uses 5- to 7-Fr guide catheters, 0.014-in guidewires, and rapid-exchange (RX) or monorail balloons and stents. These devices are manipulated by the joystick and touchscreen in cockpit. Since the range of motion of the guide catheter is only 20 cm, the target lesion must be approached manually. Once in range, lesion measurement and device deployment can be done robotically. The GRX model has several lesion crossing capabilities based on existing manual techniques. The spin function rotates the wire clockwise and counterclockwise. The rotate-on-retract is a 270-degree rotation of the wire achieved upon retraction. The wiggle function causes the wire to oscillate, to prevent prolapse in tortuous vessels. The dotter function moves

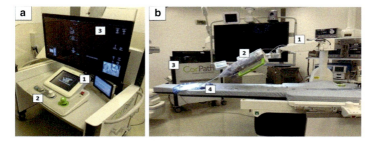

Fig. 8.3 (**a**): Workstation control, a1: touchscreen control, a2: joysticks, a3: ultra-high-definition display monitor. (**b**): Table-side robotic unit. b1: articulating arm, b2: robotic drive unit with cassette and guide catheter in place, b3: workstation. b4: in vitro flow model, cannulated with guided catheter

the wire rapidly back and forth while advancing the device which helps cross calcified lesions.

Every generation of the Corindus system is compatible with every angiogram suite and operating table. The drive is typically draped and prepared for intervention in approximately 2 minutes. The system's estimated cost is between $500,000 and $650,000, not including further single-use cassettes and devices which are approximately $300.

A primary advantage to a robotic system is the reduction of occupational hazards for the interventionalist during the robotic navigation. The technical revolution of endovascular surgery has resulted in a high volume of fluoroscopy-guided interventions, which leads to higher cumulative radiation doses for interventionalists. This has increased occupational hazards such as cataracts and left-sided neck and brain tumors [14, 15]. The journey to reduce radiation exposure paradoxically has also increased the incidence of chronic neck and spine injuries through the use of heavy leaded aprons and neck collars. By removing the operator from the direct vicinity of the radiation source, the operator can assume a more ergonomic seated position without the burden of the leaded aprons. Indeed, the RAPID II trial showed a 96.9% radiation exposure reduction for the primary interventionalist.

With robotic navigational functions, there is increased technical accuracy, eliminating physiological tremors and operative fatigue. By removing the typical movements of manual interventions, such as shaking of the hands, fast accelerations and decelerations of the devices, and unintentional wire movements or rotations during manipulations or device exchanges. This extra stability may contribute decreased technical errors and a decreased complication rate of vessel injury, distal embolization, or stent misplacement.

Telerobotic Intervention

We are on the cusp of witnessing a paradigm shift in neurovascular healthcare delivery. While not presently ready for prime time, an exciting advantage of robotic-assisted neurointervention is its ability to be performed remotely. A fully functional telerobotic endovascular system will increase access to timely, expert-performed mechanical thrombectomy for patients across the country. Mechanical thrombectomy is the standard-of-care therapy for large-vessel occlusions, but the timing of interventional treatment can dictate the clinical outcome. Presently, approximately 50% of the US population lives farther than a 60-minute drive from a thrombectomy capable site [14]. Further, geographically isolated centers with low thrombectomy volume may not be as proficient at the procedure as high-volume centers and have worse outcomes [15, 16]. As it stands, each minute of delay caused by transfer to a central location results in a 2.5% decrease in the likelihood of undergoing thrombectomy due to possibly breaching the optimal therapeutic window, ultimately rendering one-quarter of all transferred patients inoperable. If a thrombectomy can be performed at a satellite location closer to the patient, but still by the experienced neurointerventionalist, patient outcomes may improve dramatically, especially those in rural underserved areas.

This potential in remote intervention has led to proposed flow-charts for teleoperated thrombectomy by Panesar et al. [17]. In their model, non-remote intervention should still be first line and is preferable if it can be done within critical time windows. If the patient presents to a nontertiary center that has tele-thrombectomy infrastructure, a tele-consult can be performed back to the stroke team and operators at the tertiary care center. If thrombectomy is to be performed, vascular access staff (e.g., vascular surgeon, cardiologist) would obtain access, and the thrombectomy would be performed by the experienced interventionalist at the tertiary center. The patient would then be transferred to a higher-level stroke center if necessary.

Remote intervention feasibility studies have already been performed successfully in the cardiac literature. The first telerobotic PCI was described by Patel et al. in 2019 and performed with the treating cardiologist 20 miles away from the patient, utilizing the CorPath GRX [18]. Madder et al. investigated the technical requirements required for telerobotic intervention. In ex vivo and in vivo models, that group tested connection reliability and its effect on robotic-assisted interventions in a coronary artery. They found a threshold of 400 ms for perceivable latency between two sites 103 miles apart. They went further to suggest a 250 ms as a threshold for performing remote interventions. With the advent of widespread teleconferencing and the ability of many other industries to achieve two-digit millisecond latencies, undoubtedly this performance will increase. Indeed, in the first case series of five tele-PCIs, successful interventions were performed with a mean delay of 53 ms between the remote console and in suite robotic system from 20 miles [18].

The optimization and creation of distributed telerobotic thrombectomy sites may solve the issue of establishing high-cost thrombectomy centers in rural areas. Whereas the cost can be prohibitive from hiring dedicated neurointerventionalists, acquiring equipment, and ensuring 24/7 coverage, the robot may be a more efficient solution that makes the gold standard of stroke treatment available to all.

Limitations

A key limitation is the requirement of manual assistance at different stages of the intervention. The CorPath GRX is not capable of deploying devices or inflating balloons for angioplasty. A fully equivalent robotic thrombectomy would require navigation of catheters and guidewires from a femoral or radial sheath, deployment of stent retriever devices, and the ability to perform stenting or angioplasty procedures if required. Presently, a remote thrombectomy would require training the staff to deploy stent retrievers and operate aspiration peripheral devices.

Other limitations include the lack of haptic feedback during interventions. During manual procedures, catheters and wires undergo three forces which can be felt in the fingers: vicious forces between the catheter and blood, friction forces between the catheters and vessel wall, and impact forces from the tips of catheters and wires with the vessel wall. The reliance on only visual cues may theoretically increase the risk of perforations and dissections, although this has not been seen in the literature. Similarly, there is no sensory feedback on contrast administration, of which too much can potentially cause vascular injury. Regardless, remote treatment would require contingency protocols for these potential periprocedural complications such as dissection, air embolism, and access site bleeding. Further, remote intervention still requires highly trained staff and access personnel, which keeps the cost and logistical requirements of tele-thrombectomy relatively high. Other issues that arise are the cost of the systems together with the lack of randomized control trials for any of the robotic catheter systems. Further, while the primary operator is shielded from radiation, the interventional staff are still required to stay in the radiation field to change interventional equipment within the robotic arm or manually deploy devices.

Conclusions

The development and incorporation of robotic assistance into the neurointerventionalist's armamentarium is ongoing. Additional hardware and software optimizations are ongoing that will truly make the robot a practical addition to the angio suite. The near future of the robot for telerobotic thrombectomy is on the horizon and will revolutionize how we deliver equitable and highly expert stroke care.

References

1. Granada JF, Delgado JA, Uribe MP, Fernandez A, Blanco G, Leon MB, Weisz G. First-in-human evaluation of a novel robotic-assisted coronary angioplasty system. JACC Cardiovasc Interv. 2011;4(4):460–5.
2. Weisz G, Metzger DC, Caputo RP, Delgado JA, Marshall JJ, Vetrovec GW, et al. Safety and feasibility of robotic percutaneous coronary intervention: PRECISE (Percutaneous Robotically-Enhanced Coronary Intervention) Study. J Am Coll Cardiol. 2013;61(15):1596–600.
3. Mahmud E, Naghi J, Ang L, Harrison J, Behnamfar O, Pourdjabbar A, et al. Demonstration of the safety and feasibility of robotically assisted percutaneous coronary intervention in complex coronary lesions: results of the CORA-PCI Study (Complex Robotically Assisted Percutaneous Coronary Intervention). JACC Cardiovasc Interv. 2017;10(13):1320–7.

4. Mahmud E, Schmid F, Kalmar P, Deutschmann H, Hafner F, Rief P, Brodmann M. Feasibility and safety of robotic peripheral vascular interventions: results of the RAPID trial. JACC Cardiovasc Interv. 2016;9(19):2058–64.

5. Britz GW, Panesar SS, Falb P, et al. Neuroendovascular-specific engineering modifications to the CorPath GRX robotic system. J Neurosurg. 2019;1:1830–6. https://doi.org/10.3171/2019.9.JNS192113.

6. Desai VR, Lee JJ, Tomas J, Lumsden A, Britz GW. Initial experience in a pig model of robotic-assisted intracranial arteriovenous malformation (AVM) embolization. Oper Neurosurg (Hagerstown). 2020;19(2):205–9. https://doi.org/10.1093/ons/opz373. PMID: 31858149

7. Berczeli M, Chinnadurai P, Legeza PT, Britz GW, Lumsden AB. Transcarotid access for remote robotic endovascular neurointerventions: a cadaveric proof-of-concept study. Neurosurg Focus. 2022;52(1):E18. https://doi.org/10.3171/2021.10.FOCUS21511. PMID: 34973671

8. Jones B, Riga C, Bicknell C, Hamady M. Robot-assisted carotid artery stenting: a safety and feasibility study. Cardiovasc Intervent Radiol. 2021;44(5):795–800.

9. Pereira VM, Cancelliere NM, Nicholson P, et al. First-in-human, robotic-assisted neuroendovascular intervention. J Neurointerv Surg. 2020;12:338–40.

10. Cancelliere NM, Lynch J, Nicholson P, Dobrocky T, Swaminathan SK, Hendriks EJ, Krings T, Radovanovic I, Drake KE, Turner R, Sungur JM, Pereira VM. Robotic-assisted intracranial aneurysm treatment: 1 year follow-up imaging and clinical outcomes. J Neurointerv Surg. 2022;14(12):1229–33. https://doi.org/10.1136/neurintsurg-2021-017865. Epub 2021 Dec 15. PMID: 34911735; PMCID: PMC9685724

11. Desai VR, Lee JJ, Sample T, Kleiman NS, Lumsden A, Britz GW. First in man pilot feasibility study in extracranial carotid robotic-assisted endovascular intervention. Neurosurgery. 2021;88(3):506–14.

12. Sajja KC, Sweid A, Al Saiegh F, Chalouhi N, Avery MB, Schmidt RF, Tjoumakaris SI, Gooch MR, Herial N, Abbas R, Zarzour H, Romo V, Rosenwasser R, Jabbour P. Endovascular robotic: feasibility and proof of principle for diagnostic cerebral angiography and carotid artery stenting. J Neurointerv Surg. 2020;12(4):345–9. https://doi.org/10.1136/neurintsurg-2019-015763. Epub 2020 Mar 1. PMID: 32115436

13. Weinberg JH, Sweid A, Sajja K, Gooch MR, Herial N, Tjoumakaris S, Rosenwasser RH, Jabbour P. Comparison of robotic-assisted carotid stenting and manual carotid stenting through the transradial approach. J Neurosurg. 2020:1–8. https://doi.org/10.3171/2020.5.JNS201421. Epub ahead of print. PMID: 32858520

14. Brown KR, Rzucidlo E. Acute and chronic radiation injury. J Vasc Surg. 2011;53(1 Suppl):15S–21S. Reeves RR, Ang L, Bahadorani J, et al. Invasive cardiologists are exposed to greater left sided cranial

radiation: the BRAIN study (brain radiation exposure and attenuation during invasive cardiology procedures). JACC Cardiovasc Interv. 2015;8(9):1197–206.

15. Roguin A, Goldstein J, Bar O, et al. Brain and neck tumors among physicians performing interventional procedures. J Am Coll Cardiol. 2013;111(9):1368–72.

16. Adeoye O, Albright KC, Carr BG, Wolff C, Mullen MT, Abruzzo T, et al. Geographic access to acute stroke care in the United States. Stroke. 2014;45(10):3019–24.

17. Gupta R, Horev A, Nguyen T, Gandhi D, Wisco D, Glenn BA, et al. Higher volume endovascular stroke centers have faster times to treatment, higher reperfusion rates and higher rates of good clinical outcomes. J Neurointerv Surg. 2013;5(4):294–7.

18. Rinaldo L, Brinjikji W, Rabinstein AA. Transfer to high-volume centers associated with reduced mortality after endovascular treatment of acute stroke. Stroke. 2017;48(5):1316–21.

Present Rationale and Future Directions for Intracranial Aneurysm Screening and Rupture Risk Prediction: The Road to Precision Surgery for Intracranial Aneurysms

9

Abhijith R. Bathini, Maged Ghoche,
Seyed Farzad Maroufi, Brandon A. Nguyen,
Maria José Pachón-Londoño,
Ataollah Shahbandi, Devi P. Patra,
and Bernard R. Bendok

Introduction

Intracranial aneurysms (IAs) represent a significant healthcare burden due to their potential for catastrophic outcomes, including high mortality and permanent disability rates in cases of rupture. The mortality rates associated with ruptured IAs range from 23%

A. R. Bathini · M. Ghoche · M. J. Pachón-Londoño · D. P. Patra
Department of Neurological Surgery, Mayo Clinic, Phoenix, AZ, USA

Neurosurgery Simulation and Innovation Lab, Mayo Clinic,
Phoenix, AZ, USA

S. F. Maroufi · A. Shahbandi
Tehran University of Medical Sciences, Tehran, Iran

© The Author(s), under exclusive license to Springer Nature
Switzerland AG 2025
E. Veznedaroglu (ed.), *Advanced Technologies in Vascular
Neurosurgery*, https://doi.org/10.1007/978-3-031-67492-1_9

to 51%, highlighting the importance of effective screening and risk prediction strategies [1, 2]. Approximately 10% to 20% of IA rupture cases result in permanent disability, further emphasizing the critical need for early detection and intervention [1, 2]. It is therefore important to identify patients who may benefit from screening of IAs. Beyond developing appropriate screening strategies for timely detection of aneurysms, predicting risk of rupture is essential to identify patients in whom intervention may significantly reduce the likelihood of and ultimately prevent adverse events and outcomes. The use of machine learning (ML) and artificial intelligence (AI) may facilitate this process and lead to improved screening and treatment guidelines.

Overview of Major Natural History Studies

The advancement of imaging technology has transformed the detection of unruptured intracranial aneurysms (UIAs). However, our understanding of their natural evolution remains limited, sparking ongoing debates regarding their management. Over the

B. A. Nguyen
Department of Neurological Surgery, Mayo Clinic, Phoenix, AZ, USA

Neurosurgery Simulation and Innovation Lab, Mayo Clinic, Phoenix, AZ, USA

Mayo Clinic Alix School of Medicine, Scottsdale, AZ, USA

B. R. Bendok (✉)
Department of Neurological Surgery, Mayo Clinic, Phoenix, AZ, USA

Neurosurgery Simulation and Innovation Lab, Mayo Clinic, Phoenix, AZ, USA

Mayo Clinic Alix School of Medicine, Scottsdale, AZ, USA

Precision Neuro-therapeutics Innovation Lab, Mayo Clinic, Phoenix, AZ, USA

Department of Otolaryngology-Head & Neck Surgery, Mayo Clinic, Phoenix, AZ, USA

Department of Radiology, Mayo Clinic, Phoenix, AZ, USA
e-mail: Bendok.Bernard@Mayo.edu

past two decades, numerous natural history studies from around the world have been conducted, significantly shaping our strategies for evaluating and treating UIAs. However, many of these studies have significant limitations, including factors such as limited follow-up duration, sample size, and selection bias. Prospective, population-based studies are widely recognized as the gold standard for investigating the natural history of diseases, including UIAs. These studies, by observing patients over time, allow for a clearer understanding of disease progression and outcomes. Therefore, we have chosen to highlight some key prospective studies on the natural history of UIAs.

Aneurysm Rupture Risk and Predictors of Rupture

The International Study of Unruptured Intracranial Aneurysms (ISUIA 1) conducted in 1998 was a hybrid prospective and retrospective study spanning the United States, Canada, and Europe [3]. The prospective arm of the study focused on assessing treatment-related morbidity and mortality in 1172 patients with 1301 unruptured intracranial aneurysms (UIAs), followed for 1 year. The study revealed significant findings, indicating a treatment-related morbidity and mortality rate of 15.7% at 1 year. ISUIA 1 underscored the importance of factors such as aneurysm size and personal history of aneurysmal subarachnoid hemorrhage (aSAH) in assessing the management and prognosis of UIAs. It revealed that for aneurysms smaller than 10 mm, irrespective of their location, the annual rupture risk was 0.05% in patients without a history of subarachnoid hemorrhage (SAH), whereas those with a positive SAH history faced a tenfold higher risk at 0.5%. Larger aneurysms and those located at the basilar artery, vertebrobasilar or posterior cerebral artery, or posterior communicating artery were associated with a higher likelihood of rupture in patients without an SAH history. Furthermore, individuals with a family history of SAH exhibited an elevated risk of rupture particularly with basilar tip aneurysms. ISUIA 1 provided an initial comprehensive understanding of the overall rupture rate and potential predictors of aneurysm rupture in a large cohort study. Despite its extensive sample size, this study had notable limitations including follow-up period length, selection bias due to its retrospective nature, and potential confounding factors that may have influenced the results.

In 2003, the International Study of Unruptured Intracranial Aneurysms (ISUIA 2) conducted a prospective study across the United States, Canada, and Europe, involving 1692 patients with 2686 aneurysms [4]. These patients were conservatively followed for an average of 4.1 years. The study further validated the findings seen in ISUIA, including an annual rupture rate of 0.78%. Notably, in individuals with no history of aneurysmal subarachnoid hemorrhage (aSAH), aneurysms in internal carotid, anterior communicating, anterior cerebral, or middle cerebral arteries had a rupture rate of 0% for those smaller than 7 mm, 2.6% for 7–12 mm, 14.5% for 13–24 mm, and 40% for 25 mm or larger. In contrast, for aneurysms in the posterior circulation and posterior communicating artery, the rates were slightly higher: 2.5%, 14.5%, 18.4%, and 50%, respectively, for the same size categories. Predictors of rupture identified in the study included aneurysm size, location (particularly involving the posterior circulation or posterior communicating artery), and a history of aSAH. However, the study encountered limitations, notably selection bias and a high dropout rate, which may have impacted the generalizability of the findings [4]. It should be noted that the low rupture rate for small anterior circulation aneurysms has remained controversial in light of the fact that anterior communicating artery aneurysms are most seen clinically and their median size of rupture is 7 mm.

ISUIA I and II provide initial perspectives into the natural history of unruptured intracranial aneurysms. Subsequent studies have further enriched our understanding of UIA behavior and response to treatment. Ishibashi et al. (2009) followed 419 patients with 529 unruptured aneurysms for 2.5 years [5]. Their findings were consistent with previous studies, further highlighting the role of size (>10 mm), location (posterior circulation), and history of subarachnoid hemorrhage in aneurysm rupture, with an annual rupture rate of 1.4%. Similarly, Lee et al. (2012), after following

5963 patients conservatively for 3.3 years, reported an annual rupture rate of 2.7% [6]. In their study, only age was significantly associated with rupture. However, this study notably failed to report important data, such as UIA morphology, location, and size, which could help identify risk factors. They claimed that their aim only focused on the incidence of aneurysm rupture in the untreated group and UIA treatment.

The Unruptured Cerebral Aneurysm Study of Japan (UCAS) [7], conducted in 2012, offered substantial insights into the natural history and treatment outcomes of UIAs. With an annual rupture rate of 0.95%, UIAs larger than 7 mm, located in the posterior or anterior communicating arteries, were associated with a higher rate of rupture. Unlike previous studies, UCAS was the first to provide a correlation between morphology, specifically the presence of a daughter sac defined as an irregular protrusion in the wall of the aneurysm, and the risk of rupture. Surprisingly, according to this study, a history of subarachnoid hemorrhage, family history, and smoking were not identified as potential risk factors. UCAS study faced several limitations, including a high dropout rate for aneurysms treated during the follow-up period, a homogenous study population, and potential selection bias.

It is imperative to recognize the profound impact that the aforementioned studies have had on clinical decision-making regarding the optimal care for patients diagnosed with unruptured intracranial aneurysms. These studies have significantly contributed to enhancing our understanding of the management strategies and outcomes associated with this complex condition. However, it is essential to emphasize a common limitation shared among these studies: the relatively short follow-up periods. While follow-ups ranging from 1 to 4 years can provide valuable insights into the progression and management of intracranial aneurysms over the short term, extending these follow-up durations could offer even deeper insights. Prolonged follow-up periods exceeding the conventional 1–4 years window will allow comprehensive data extraction regarding the natural history of aneurysms. By tracking the evolution of aneurysms over extended periods, we can obtain more accurate assessments of rupture rates, long-term posttreatment complications, and the stability of aneurysms in terms of size, morphology, and rupture risk. Moreover, longer follow-up durations enable clinicians to observe the durability of treatment interventions and their sustained effects on aneurysm stability and patient outcomes.

One good example is the Finnish study published in 2013 by Juvela et al. [8]. Although they had a small sample size (142 patients), their median follow-up time was 21 years, long enough to provide reliable and consistent data on the evolution of these aneurysms. Juvela reported an annual rupture rate of 1.1%, with smoking, anterior location, size (≥ 7 mm), and inversely the age as predictors of hemorrhage. In addition, because of their long follow-up period, they discovered that the annual risk of bleeding increased with age. This longitudinal perspective study is invaluable in refining treatment protocols, optimizing patient care pathways, and informing evidence-based clinical guidelines. Therefore, while the existing studies have undoubtedly advanced our understanding of unruptured intracranial aneurysms, future research endeavors should prioritize extended follow-up periods to provide a more comprehensive understanding of the disease trajectory and optimize patient management strategies.

Familial Aneurysms

The term familial intracranial aneurysm (FIA) refers to the presence of proven aneurysms in at least two first-degree relatives. In 1954, Chambers et al. published the first report on a familial aggregation of IAs [9]. Since then many studies investigating familial aggregation of intracranial aneurysms (IAs) have been published, offering insights into the underlying mechanisms driving IA pathogenesis, rupture, and familial clustering.

Approximately 10% of subarachnoid hemorrhage (SAH) patients exhibit a familial history of IAs, with the first-degree relatives facing a 2.5- to 7-fold increased odds of experiencing aneurysmal SAH compared to the general population [10, 11]. Additionally, across various ethnic groups, the prevalence of familial history remains equal, with rates of 19.4%, 20.6%, and 21.6% among Caucasian, African American, and Hispanic patients with IAs, respectively [12].

The familial aggregation observed in FIA families, along with the absence of concurrent disorders predisposing them to IA, points to the notion that certain IAs may possess a distinct genetic component independent of previously defined diseases (i.e., ADPKD, Ehlers Danlos, Loeys-Dietz, etc.). This hypothesis is reinforced by recent DNA linkage studies, which have identified potential genetic loci associated with cerebral aneurysms, such as 19q in the Finnish population and 7q11 in the Japanese population, based on sibling-pair analyses [13, 14]. Moreover, to further elucidate the genetic underpinnings of FIAs, a whole-genome linkage study utilizing over 5000 single nucleotide polymorphisms (SNPs) revealed potential evidence of linkage to chromosomes 4, 7, 8, and 12, with indications of a possible gene-smoking interaction on chromosomes 4, 7, and 12 [15]. In addition, the concept of anticipation, initially proposed in Dutch studies, has been observed in FIAs [16]. These studies suggested a trend of FIA ruptures occurring at earlier ages in successive generations, hinting at a potential genetic basis for the observed phenomenon. However, subsequent research has found controversial results, highlighting the influence of variables such as the length of follow-up and the inclusion of asymptomatic cases in shaping familial IA trends [17]. It should be noted that the presence of anticipation, while intriguing, may complicate the search for specific genetic markers through genome-wide screens, underscoring the need for more advanced and delicate approaches to dissect the genetic underpinnings of familial IA.

Studies examining familial aggregation consistently point toward distinct clinical characteristics of FIAs compared to sporadic cases. Familial aneurysms tend to rupture earlier and are smaller in size, suggesting potential differences in the underlying pathophysiology [18, 19]. Geometric and morphological risk factors for IA rupture are comparable between familial and sporadic ruptured aneurysms, suggesting the presence of additional unidentified risk factors in FIA cases [20]. Moreover, aneurysm size at rupture within familial IAs has demonstrated a lack of concordance, suggesting that the size of a ruptured IA in one family member may not significantly influence the management of an unruptured IA in another relative [21]. Interestingly, aneurysms in siblings frequently rupture within the same decade of life, highlighting potential shared temporal vulnerabilities [22].

Familial cases exhibit a predilection for certain anatomical locations, such as the anterior communicating artery complex, and are associated with a higher incidence of multiple and de novo aneurysms [23]. Moreover, in a well-selected cohort with familial susceptibility to IA development, there was greater territorial concordance of IAs when comparing probands with their affected first-degree relatives than with unrelated patients, implying a predisposition to IA formation based on anatomical factors [24]. Future investigations into IA genetics should consider stratifying cases by IA location, recognizing the role of heritable structural vulnerability in influencing IA multiplicity and distribution.

The overall mortality rates are similar between affected and unaffected individuals in families with FIAs. Meanwhile, those with ruptured IAs experienced higher mortality rates compared to those without rupture, underscoring the critical importance of preventing IA rupture in affected individuals [25]. To prevent rupture, timely diagnosis of aneurysms is crucial in patients with FIAs. Brown et al. have suggested screening for familial aneurysms to be performed among the affected patients' first-degree relatives who have known risk factors for IA development, including older age (>30 years), female gender, and a history of smoking (20-pack-year smoking) or hypertension (for at least 10 years) [26]. Notably, Leblanc et al. proposed an optimal age for angiographic screening in individuals at risk of familial SAH, recommending ages 20–53.5 years for women and 20–49 years for men [27]. Additionally, Raaymakers et al. suggested that siblings of familial SAH patients are most at risk of unruptured aneurysm compared to the children of the patients [28]. Accordingly, the screening for unruptured IAs should be targeted to these specific individuals. The cost-effectiveness of targeted screening in patients susceptible to FIAs has been established in the study by Takao et al., suggesting magnetic resonance angiography in older family members with two or more affected first-degree relatives [29].

Autosomal Dominant Polycystic Kidney Disease

Certain genetic disorders, such as type IV Ehlers-Danlos syndrome, Marfan syndrome, Loeys-Dietz syndrome, and autosomal dominant polycystic kidney disease (ADPKD), have been found to significantly increase the risk of intracranial aneurysm formation [30, 31]. ADPKD is the most common hereditary kidney disorder with a prevalence of 1:1000 live births [32, 33]. While characterized by the development of multiple cysts in the kidneys, ADPKD is associated with multiple extrarenal complications such as hepatic and pancreatic cysts and hypertension. IA occurrence in ADPKD patients has been assessed in several random screening studies which have typically reported a prevalence of 9–14, representing a three- to fivefold increase compared to the general population [34, 35]. A 2017 meta-analysis on IA prevalence, risk factors, and natural history in asymptomatic ADPKD patients by Zhou et al. found a prevalence of 10% (95% CI 7–13) [36]. A 1998 meta-analysis by Rinkel et al. reported an IA prevalence in ADPKD patients undergoing angiographic studies of 10% (95% CI 6.2–15%) [37]. A 2011 meta-analysis on UIA prevalence by Vlak et al. found a prevalence ratio of 6.9 for ADPKD patients compared to patients without ADPKD [34]. The heterogeneity of the prevalence calculated in this meta-analysis was high, likely due to the inclusion of studies with smaller sample sizes and inconsistency between selection criteria between studies but also potentially due to differences intrinsic to patient populations in different geographic regions.

In ADPKD patients, IAs also tend to develop earlier and with a higher risk of rupture compared to the general population, with a mean age of rupture of 41 (compared to 51 in the general population) [38, 39]. Several hypotheses have been proposed for the increased incidence and risk of rupture of IA in ADPKD patients, with endothelial dysfunction and increased circulating inflammatory markers being most often implicated. Most cases of ADPKD are attributable to mutations in *PKD1* and *PKD2*, genes coding the proteins polycystin-1 and polycystin-2, respectively [32, 33, 40]. These proteins are implicated in maintaining vascular structural integrity, and in murine models, homozygous mutations in either *PKD1* or *PKD2* resulted in embryonic death with increased vascular fragility [41, 42].

While a personal or familial history of unruptured IAs or SAH is a recognized risk factor in individuals with ADPKD, additional risk factors, such as sex, hypertension, smoking, kidney disease progression, and genetic predisposition associated with specific ethnic origins such as Chinese, Japanese, German, or Polish ethnicity, may further augment risk of IA development but have not been as well established [36, 38, 43–45]. Zhou et al. also assessed risk factors in their 2017 meta-analysis, reporting statistically significant increased risk associated with family history of IA/SAH (RR = 2.33, 95% CI 1.60, 3.38). However, this meta-analysis did not identify sex, smoking, hypertension, age, or renal dysfunction (defined as stage 3–5 CKD) as significant risk factors [36]. Regarding associations between kidney function and IA detection, a study on ADPKD patients in Japan undergoing periodic universal screening published by Kataoka et al. in 2022 found that total kidney volume (TKV) $\geq$ 1000 mL, height-adjusted TKV $\geq$ 500 mL, Mayo imaging classification classes 1D–1E, and chronic kidney disease stages 3–5 were significantly associated with increased risk for IA [45]. In a separate study on genetic risk factors, Kataoka et al. also found associations between splicing and frameshift mutation types with IA in ADPKD patients [44].

Universal versus selective screening for IA in the ADPKD population is a subject of debate. In 2015, the KDIGO conference discouraged universal IA screening in ADPKD patients for similar reasons as the general population [40]. While some providers do universally screen for IA at time of ADPKD diagnosis, screening is more often performed on an individual basis based on a shared decision-making process, with routine screening only performed in patients with ADPKD and history of prior aneurysm rupture, family history of SAH or IA, high-risk occupations (such as pilots), or prior high-risk non-emergent surgeries (such as kidney transplantation) [38, 40]. A 2018 single-center study on 495 consecutive ADPKD patients published by Flahault et al. assessed two groups—one with family history of IA and one without family history of IA—and reported imaging results, management, rate of rupture, and outcomes. The authors performed a cost-utility analysis which suggested that a universal screening strategy may be more cost-effective and reduce occurrence of IA rupture and IA-associated death when compared to screening only patients with a family history of IA/SAH and no screening [46].

Considering the high morbidity and mortality associated with ruptured IA even with appropriate intervention and the absence of consensus regarding the selection criteria for screening ADPKD patients, there is a necessity to determine the specific subset of ADPKD patients who should undergo screening for IA. Future prospective, multicenter trials will be needed to shed more light on this subject.

Present Guidelines for Screening Unruptured Intracranial Aneurysms

Based on a number of natural history studies, including some listed in the previous sections, certain screening guidelines have been developed which will be explored in this section. Screening strategies should be determined on a case-by-case basis, considering individual patient risk factors [47]. For tailoring the optimal screening plan, the prevalence of intracranial aneurysms (IAs) associated with the patient's condition(s), estimated IA morbidity, availability of a cost-effective modality for screening, and accessibility to safe and efficacious treatment should be weighed against the patient's stress and anxiety resulting from detecting an IA [48, 49].

According to the latest American Heart Association (AHA) guidelines, MR angiography and CT angiography are recommended for screening as noninvasive imaging modalities [50]. The guidelines outline four indications for screening, with level B evidence (Table 9.1) [50]:

Table 9.1 Guidelines outline four indications for screening, with level B evidence

Class I recommendations
Patients with ≥ 2 family members with IAs or a history of SAH with a particularly elevated risk of aneurysm occurrence in patients with a history of hypertension, smoking, or of the female sex
Patients with a history of ADPKD, especially in patients with a positive family history regarding IAs
Class IIa recommendations
Patients with a history of coarctation of aorta
Patients with microcephalic osteodysplastic primordial dwarfism

Newly Investigated Correlations to Aneurysm Prevalence

Following 2015 AHA guidelines, various new comorbidities and diseases have been investigated as possible novel indications for screening:

- *Tobacco consumption and female gender.* Recent literature has shown that the combination of female sex and tobacco consumption may considerably increase the prevalence of IAs [51–56]. Ogilvy et al. performed a multicenter case-control study on middle-aged women aged 30–60 using MRA to assess whether smoking conferred an increased risk of having an unruptured IA. The authors discovered that women with a positive smoking history demonstrated a fourfold higher risk of having an unruptured IA. This correlation increased to seven-fold if the patients had underlying chronic hypertension. Hence, screening for IAs in this population may offer clinical utility. The group then further performed a cost-effective analysis in this patient group based on various screening strategies. Of the 30 different screening strategies that were trialed, all of them yielded extra quality-adjusted life years, with screening at a younger age conferring more health benefit at a lower cost. Furthermore, all models had a significant impact on prevention of subarachnoid hemorrhage [56].

- *First-degree relatives of patients with a history of IA.* Van Hoe at el. performed a meta-analysis of 37 articles assessing the utility of screening for IAs in patients with positive first-degree family history [57]. The authors reported that individuals with ≥2 affected first-degree relatives had a 13.1% prevalence of IA, while the prevalence in the general population was only 3%. There is general consensus that screening is cost-effective and recommended in this particular group. In contrast, individuals with ≥1 affected first-degree relatives had a lower average prevalence of having an IA at 4.8%. Although screening IAs in this group may be cost-effective, present evidence suggests that the need for screening for this group of individuals should be adjudicated on a case-by-case basis, as the prevalence of IAs may vary greatly based on the presence of other risk factors [56–58].
- *Connective tissue disorders.* A large study from Mayo Clinic evaluated the prevalence of IAs in the context of various connective tissue disorders over a 10-year time period. They identified the prevalence of IAs in these patient groups as follows: 28% in Loeys-Dietz syndrome, 14% in Marfan syndrome, 12% in Ehlers-Danlos syndrome, and 11% in neurofibromatosis type 1 [59]. Other studies have largely corroborated these findings while alluding to other potential connective tissue disorders that may correlate with a higher risk of IA formation such as osteogenesis imperfecta [31, 60–63].

There has been some previous speculation that hereditary hemorrhagic telangiectasia (HHT) can be associated with the formation of IAs due to hemodynamic flow abnormalities in the cerebral vasculature. However, present evidence does not support this hypothesis. The prevalence of IAs appears similar between patients with HHT and the general population [64, 65]. On the other hand, due to hyperdynamic flow, sporadic AVMs are highly associated with aneurysms [66]. A similar theory may have also existed with patients who have a history of Kawasaki disease [67–69]. Although inflammation has a key role in the formation of

IAs and the pathogenesis of Kawasaki disease, and there have been comparable histopathological findings in the two conditions [67, 68], present definitive evidence does not support the suggestion of an association between these two pathologic entities [69].

Various studies have also pointed out other diseases and pathologies that potentially correlate with a higher prevalence of IAs. It is important to note that many of these studies listed below contain a limited subset of patients that may not represent the broader population. Further population-based studies will be required for validation before true conclusions can be made and before screening protocols can be developed based on these variables:

- *Patients with low ankle-brachial index (ABI)*. A group from Finland assessed the link between IAs and low ABI, which has been associated with an elevated risk of cardiovascular events. Nearly 3000 patients were included with ABI measurements. Of these, 776 patients had available cerebrovascular imaging or an IA diagnosis. After dividing these patients based on ABI severity, their results showed that the prevalence of IAs was 20.3% in the low ABI group, 14.9% in the borderline ABI group, 7.0% in the high ABI group, and 2.4% in the normal ABI group. Overall, the prevalence of unruptured IAs was nearly ninefold higher in the low ABI group when compared to the normal ABI group [70].
- *Patients with a history of sellar lesions*. Yan et al. aimed to evaluate the coexistence of IAs and sellar lesions within the Chinese population. A total of 405 consecutive patients were included in the study, of which 45 patients were concurrently diagnosed with IAs by CTA, DSA, or intraoperative findings. The authors concluded that, in their study, the overall prevalence IAs in patients with sellar lesions was as high as 11.1%, which is higher than previous studies of the Chinese population that reported a prevalence ranging from 1% to 8% [71].
- *Patients with late-onset Pompe disease (LOPD)*. Multiple studies report a higher incidence of IAs in patients affected by LOPD. The disease process involves periodic acid-Schiff

(PAS)-positive vacuoles indicating abnormal glycogen storage inside the smooth muscle cells of the intracranial arteries. This pathology may alter the normal architecture of the vessel wall, thereby possibly leading to IA formation [72]. In an analysis of a cohort of 52 patients representing the Belgian population, two patients were found to have IAs, while another two were found to have vertebrobasilar dolichoectasia [73]. In another study of 21 patients involving the Italian population, 14% of patients were found to have unruptured IAs, while nearly 50% of the patients had vertebrobasilar dolichoectasia [74, 75].

- *Patients with fibromuscular dysplasia (FMD).* Noninflammatory and non-atherosclerotic changes of the arteries in FMD are most classically known to target renal and cervical arteries [59, 77]. It is postulated that intracranial arteries may be affected as well, thereby leading to IA formation. Based on a review of 669 women from the US Registry for FMD, the authors found that the prevalence of IAs in patients with FMD is approximately 13% [76–79].

- *Patients with sickle cell disease.* In a study of almost 250 patients with sickle cell disease, routine screening using MRA was performed. Authors of the study reported a prevalence of IAs at 11% in these patients [80]. This could possibly be due to vessel wall dilation caused by endothelial dysfunction and disruption of elastic lamina [81, 82].

- *Patients with a history of systemic atherosclerosis.* A correlation between systemic atherosclerosis and IAs has been suggested in the literature [83]. A retrospective case-control study involving approximately 1700+ patients from Finland revealed that abdominal aortic calcification is greater in both ruptured and unruptured IAs. This could be due to the fact that inflammation of the vessel wall is a major contributor to both IA formation and atherosclerosis [61, 84].

- *Patients with a history of transient ischemic attack (TIA) or ischemic stroke.* Present literature demonstrates that 4.7–12.4% of patients with a history of TIA or ischemic stroke may have previously unknown, asymptomatic unruptured IAs [85–87]. This finding may be explained by the fact that TIA/ischemic stroke and IA formation have some shared risk factors such as hypertension and smoking [61].

- *Patients with aortopathies or extracranial arteriopathies.* This is a broad topic involving many pathologies. One example is a bicuspid aortic valve. Multiple studies report that patients with bicuspid aortic valves may have a higher prevalence of IAs ranging from 7.7% to 8% [88–91]. Another example is that patients with a history of aortic aneurysm and/or dissection also have a higher prevalence of IAs ranging from 6.8% to 23% across various studies [92–95]. Furthermore, up to 25.7% of patients with renal artery aneurysms may harbor IAs [96, 97]. Additionally, 23% of patients with spontaneous coronary artery dissection may have at least one IA [98]. There are many possibilities as to why these correlations exist, but it is possible that these pathologies share a genetic predisposition to vascular fragility. Moreover, hypertension may also be an underlying factor in their pathogenesis [61].

Table 9.2 summarizes the findings of this section:

Table 9.2 Newly investigated correlations to aneurysm prevalence	**Novel indications for screening with strong evidence**
	Tobacco consumption and female gender
	First-degree relatives of patients with a history of IA
	Connective tissue disorders
	Associations with limited evidence
	Low ankle-brachial index (ABI)
	History of sellar lesions
	Late-onset Pompe disease (LOPD)
	Fibromuscular dysplasia (FMD)
	Sickle cell disease
	Systemic atherosclerosis
	History of transient ischemic attack (TIA) or ischemic stroke
	Aortopathies or extracranial arteriopathies

Future Directions for Screening of Intracranial Aneurysms

The present guidelines for screening are based on population studies in which overall rates of IA prevalence, incidence, growth, rupture, and mortality were reported in a heterogeneous population [99–103]. However, as medicine moves toward individualized care, it becomes necessary to tailor the screening strategy specifically to each patient. To this end, it is critical to adopt a holistic approach that considers demographic characteristics such as age, sex, and race, comorbidities such as hypertension and smoking, and individual genetics such as histories of connective tissue disorders, genetic syndromes, and familial IAs. To develop such strategies, we need data from prospective studies with long-term follow-up, along with assistance from artificial intelligence and machine learning algorithms [99–103].

Artificial Intelligence in Aneurysm Screening

Artificial intelligence has great potential to enhance patient care. Several studies have utilized AI models as a tool for screening IA development. Heo et al. utilized a comprehensive dataset derived from the National Health Screening Program in Korea to develop ML models predicting the presence of IA [101]. The ML models reported the risk of IA development on a quantile scale. The study found an AUROC of 0.75 and higher across different AI models, revealing the effectiveness of such a tool in predicting the risk of aneurysm development. Moreover, the risk stratifications retrieved from the ML models were associated with the patient's survival. These findings underscore the potential utility of the developed prediction model in guiding future IA screening strategies, facilitating early detection and intervention among high-risk individuals. This innovative approach holds promise for enhancing IA management protocols, ultimately contributing to improved patient outcomes and resource utilization efficiency in healthcare settings.

AI has gained interest as a novel tool for improving the accuracy of aneurysm risk prediction. Machine learning (ML) and deep learning (DL) algorithms have been established to have superior performance in predicting various medical outcomes compared to human assessors and conventional statistical models. Regarding the two algorithms, ML algorithms rely on pre-extracted features from input data, while DL algorithms utilize neural networks to analyze complex datasets [104]. In the context of aneurysm risk assessment, AI models can integrate various types of data, including basic clinical information, morphological data, and hemodynamic variables, to generate accurate predictions. AI-based prediction models have shown encouraging results in enhancing the efficacy of aneurysm risk assessment by identifying subtle patterns and relationships that may not be apparent. The main challenges in aneurysm risk assessment revolve around the intricate and entangled relationships between various predictive factors [105].

In recent years, the application of AI in rupture risk prediction has gained more and more interest. A number of publications have investigated different AI modes based on various input data to optimize the risk of rupture prediction. Among these publications, AI has reportedly outperformed conventional statistical models, human assessors, and the PHASES score. In 2007, Lau et al. reported an initial experience with AI models to predict the risk of rupture [106]. They reported their experience and challenges in developing an ensemble model based on highly unbalanced data with many missing values, as is often observed in many clinical settings. Ensemble models are believed to reach higher performance indices by optimally combining the predictions from multiple individual AI models. Kim et al. devised a convolutional neural network (CNN) based on 3D digital subtraction angiography (DSA) images, focusing on 368 anterior circulation aneurysms smaller than 7 mm [107]. They demonstrated that the diagnostic accuracy of the CNN model surpassed that of human assessors (AUROC of 0.755 vs. 0.537; $p < 0.001$). Moreover, in a study by Zhu et al., comprising a cohort of 2076 aneurysms, various clinical and morphological characteristics were compared using different ML models [108]. These ML models were com-

Table 9.3 Key morphological parameters

Key morphological parameters
Maximum diameter, neck diameter, maximum height
Aneurysm angle, inflow angle, branching angle
Presence of daughter sac, multiple lobes
Aspect ratio (ratio of maximum height to neck diameter)
Size ratio (ratio of maximum diameter to parent vessel diameter)
Parent vessel diameters, proximal and distal to aneurysm
Ellipticity index, undulation index, non-sphericity index

pared with those of traditional logistic regression and the PHASES score, aiming to predict the rupture status of the aneurysm. They revealed that the AI models (with AUROC ranging from 0.831 to 0.851) significantly outperformed the conventional logistic regression model (0.810, $p = 0.038$) and the PHASES score (0.615, $p < 0.01$).

Many of these models have traditionally been synthesized based on morphological characteristics, including some of the key parameters listed in Table 9.3 [109–111]:

Transcending beyond these traditional parameters, the burgeoning utilization of computational fluid dynamics (CFD) within AI models represents a paradigm shift in the assessment of aneurysm rupture risk. Unlike traditional approaches that primarily rely on morphological and baseline characteristics, AI models incorporating CFD data may offer enhanced efficacy in predicting aneurysm rupture. By simulating blood flow dynamics within the aneurysm sac, CFD-based AI models can capture intricate hemodynamic features that are pivotal in determining the likelihood of rupture. These models provide a more comprehensive understanding of the underlying biomechanical factors contributing to aneurysm progression, enabling more accurate risk stratification. Shi et al. investigated the rupture risk for small aneurysms identified through computed tomography angiography and invasive cerebral angiography [112]. They developed various ML models and compared the diagnostic efficacy of clinical, morphological, and hemodynamic data as input for models. Analysis of various input data revealed that hemodynamic parameters were the most predictive indicators of aneurysm rupture risk. The study found no significant difference between internal and external validation datasets, underscoring the reliability and generalizability of the model across different clinical settings. The trend reflected in the latter study and many others demonstrate a growing recognition of the importance of dynamic hemodynamic parameters in predicting aneurysm behavior and signify a shift toward personalized and precision medicine approaches in the management of cerebral aneurysms [113, 114].

Conclusions

Screening for intracranial aneurysms and rupture risk prediction are dynamic topics of discussion. Many natural history studies have paved the way for the guidelines that are presently in place. The limitations inherent within these studies, however, will hopefully be tackled by high-quality prospective studies which incorporate modern AI tools. These studies will hopefully be enhanced in the context of groundbreaking genomics research along with revolutionary advancements in artificial intelligence and machine learning. Together, these innovations facilitate unparalleled data extraction and analysis with the ultimate goal of improving and optimizing patient outcomes as we move toward the era of precision surgery in the care of intracranial aneurysms.

References

1. Macdonald RL, Schweizer TA. Spontaneous subarachnoid hemorrhage. Lancet. 2017;389(10069):655–66.
2. Ingall T, Asplund K, Mähönen M, Bonita R. A multinational comparison of subarachnoid hemorrhage epidemiology in the WHO MONICA stroke study. Stroke. 2000;31(5):1054–61.
3. International Study of Unruptured Intracranial Aneurysms Investigators. Unruptured intracranial aneurysms—risk of rupture and risks of surgical intervention. N Engl J Med. 1998;339:1725–33.

 4. Wiebers DO, Whisnant JP, Huston J 3rd, Meissner I, Brown RD Jr, Piepgras DG, et al. Unruptured intracranial aneurysms: natural history, clinical outcome, and risks of surgical and endovascular treatment. Lancet. 2003;362:103–10.

 5. Ishibashi T, Murayama Y, Urashima M, Saguchi T, Ebara M, Arakawa H, Irie K, Takao H, Abe T. Unruptured intracranial aneurysms: incidence of rupture and risk factors. Stroke. 2009;40(1):313–6. https://doi.org/10.1161/STROKEAHA.108.521674.

 6. Lee EJ, Lee HJ, Hyun MK, Choi JE, Kim JH, Lee NR, Hwang JS, Kwon JW. Rupture rate for patients with untreated unruptured intracranial aneurysms in South Korea during 2006-2009. J Neurosurg. 2012;117(1):53–9. https://doi.org/10.3171/2012.3.JNS111221.

 7. Investigators UJ, Morita A, Kirino T, Hashi K, Aoki N, Fukuhara S, et al. The natural course of unruptured cerebral aneurysms in a Japanese cohort. N Engl J Med. 2012;366:2474–82.

 8. Juvela S, Poussa K, Lehto H, Porras M. Natural history of unruptured intracranial aneurysms: a long-term follow-up study. Stroke. 2013;44(9):2414–2421. https://doi.org/10.1161/STROKEAHA. 113.001838.

 9. Chambers WR, Harper BF Jr, Simpson JR. Familial incidence of congenital aneurysms of cerebral arteries: report of cases of ruptured aneurysms in father and son. JAMA J Am Med Assoc. 1954;155(4):358–9.

10. Bor AS, Rinkel GJ, Adami J, Koffijberg H, Ekbom A, Buskens E, et al. Risk of subarachnoid haemorrhage according to number of affected relatives: a population based case-control study. Brain. 2008;131(Pt 10):2662–5.

11. Leblanc R. Familial cerebral aneurysms. Can J Neurol Sci. 1997;24(3):191–9.

12. Kim DH, Van Ginhoven G, Milewicz DM. Incidence of familial intracranial aneurysms in 200 patients: comparison among Caucasian, African-American, and Hispanic populations. Neurosurgery. 2003;53(2):302–8.

13. Olson JM, Vongpunsawad S, Kuivaniemi H, Ronkainen A, Hernesniemi J, Ryynänen M, et al. Search for intracranial aneurysm susceptibility gene(s) using Finnish families. BMC Med Genet. 2002;3:7.

14. Onda H, Kasuya H, Yoneyama T, Takakura K, Hori T, Takeda J, et al. Genomewide-linkage and haplotype-association studies map intracranial aneurysm to chromosome 7q11. Am J Hum Genet. 2001;69(4):804–19.

15. Foroud T, Sauerbeck L, Brown R, Anderson C, Woo D, Kleindorfer D, et al. Genome screen to detect linkage to intracranial aneurysm susceptibility genes: the Familial Intracranial Aneurysm (FIA) study. Stroke. 2008;39(5):1434–40.

16. Ruigrok YM, Rinkel GJ, Wijmenga C, Van Gijn J. Anticipation and phenotype in familial intracranial aneurysms. J Neurol Neurosurg Psychiatry. 2004;75(10):1436–42.

17. Woo D, Hornung R, Sauerbeck L, Brown R, Meissner I, Huston J, et al. Age at intracranial aneurysm rupture among generations: Familial Intracranial Aneurysm Study. Neurology. 2009;72(8):695–8.

18. Bromberg JE, Rinkel GJ, Algra A, Limburg M, van Gijn J. Outcome in familial subarachnoid hemorrhage. Stroke. 1995;26(6):961–3.

19. Lindgaard L, Eskesen V, Gjerris F, Olsen NV. Familial aggregation of intracranial aneurysms in an Inuit patient population in Kalaallit Nunaat (Greenland). Neurosurgery. 2003;52(2):357–62; discussion 62–3

20. Mensing LA, Rinkel GJ, Vlak MH, van der Schaaf IC, Ruigrok YM. Difference in aneurysm characteristics between patients with familial and sporadic aneurysmal subarachnoid haemorrhage. PloS One. 2016;11(4):e0154281.

21. Bourcier R, Lindgren A, Desal H, L'Allinec V, Januel AC, Koivisto T, et al. Concordance in aneurysm size at time of rupture in familial intracranial aneurysms. Stroke. 2019;50(2):504–6.

22. Kasuya H, Onda H, Takeshita M, Hori T, Takakura K. Clinical features of intracranial aneurysms in siblings. Neurosurgery. 2000;46(6):1301–5; discussion 5–6

23. ter Berg HW, Dippel DW, Limburg M, Schievink WI, van Gijn J. Familial intracranial aneurysms. A review. Stroke. 1992;23(7):1024–30.

24. Mackey J, Brown RD Jr, Moomaw CJ, Hornung R, Sauerbeck L, Woo D, et al. Familial intracranial aneurysms: is anatomic vulnerability heritable? Stroke. 2013;44(1):38–42.

25. Sauerbeck L, Hornung R, Woo D, Moomaw C, Anderson C, Connolly E, et al. Mortality and causes of death in the familial intracranial aneurysm study. Int J Stroke. 2012:8.

26. Brown RD Jr, Huston J, Hornung R, Foroud T, Kallmes DF, Kleindorfer D, et al. Screening for brain aneurysm in the Familial Intracranial Aneurysm Study: frequency and predictors of lesion detection. J Neurosurg. 2008;108(6):1132–8.

27. Leblanc R, Worsley KJ, Melanson D, Tampieri D. Angiographic screening and elective surgery of familial cerebral aneurysms: a decision analysis. Neurosurgery. 1994;35(1):9–18.

28. Raaymakers TW, Rinkel GJ, Ramos LM. Initial and follow-up screening for aneurysms in families with familial subarachnoid hemorrhage. Neurology. 1998;51(4):1125–30.

29. Takao H, Nojo T, Ohtomo K. Screening for familial intracranial aneurysms: decision and cost-effectiveness analysis. Acad Radiol. 2008;15(4):462–71.

30. Brown R. Unruptured intracranial aneurysms. Semin Neurol. 2010;30(05):537–44. https://doi.org/10.1055/s-0030-1268858.

31. Kim JH, Kim JW, Song SW, et al. Intracranial aneurysms are associated with Marfan syndrome. Stroke. 2021;52(1):331–4. https://doi.org/10.1161/STROKEAHA.120.032107.

32. Cornec-Le Gall E, Alam A, Perrone RD. Autosomal dominant polycystic kidney disease. Lancet. 2019;393(10174):919–35. https://doi.org/10.1016/S0140-6736(18)32782-X.

33. Rastogi A, Ameen KM, Al-Baghdadi M, et al. Autosomal dominant polycystic kidney disease: updated perspectives. Ther Clin Risk Manag. 2019;15:1041–52. https://doi.org/10.2147/TCRM.S196244.

34. Vlak MH, Algra A, Brandenburg R, Rinkel GJ. Prevalence of unruptured intracranial aneurysms, with emphasis on sex, age, comorbidity, country, and time period: a systematic review and meta-analysis. Lancet Neurol. 2011;10(7):626–36. https://doi.org/10.1016/S1474-4422(11)70109-0.

35. Capelli I, Zoli M, Righini M, et al. MR brain screening in ADPKD patients. Clin Neuroradiol. 2022;32(1):69–78. https://doi.org/10.1007/s00062-021-01050-0.

36. Zhou Z, Xu Y, Delcourt C, et al. Is regular screening for intracranial aneurysm necessary in patients with autosomal dominant polycystic kidney disease? A systematic review and meta-analysis. Cerebrovasc Dis. 2017;44(1–2):75–82. https://doi.org/10.1159/000476073.

37. Rinkel GJE, Djibuti M, Algra A, van Gijn J. Prevalence and risk of rupture of intracranial aneurysms. Stroke. 1998;29(1):251–6. https://doi.org/10.1161/01.STR.29.1.251.

38. Sanchis IM, Shukoor S, Irazabal MV, et al. Presymptomatic screening for intracranial aneurysms in patients with autosomal dominant polycystic kidney disease. Clin J Am Soc Nephrol. 2019;14(8):1151–60. https://doi.org/10.2215/CJN.14691218.

39. Chauveau D, Pirson Y, Verellen-Dumoulin C, Macnicol A, Gonzalo A, Grünfeld JP. Intracranial aneurysms in autosomal dominant polycystic kidney disease. Kidney Int. 1994;45(4):1140–6. https://doi.org/10.1038/ki.1994.151.

40. Chapman AB, Devuyst O, Eckardt KU, et al. Autosomal-dominant polycystic kidney disease (ADPKD): executive summary from a Kidney Disease: Improving Global Outcomes (KDIGO) controversies conference. Kidney Int. 2015;88(1):17–27. https://doi.org/10.1038/ki.2015.59.

41. Kim K, Drummond I, Ibraghimov-Beskrovnaya O, Klinger K, Arnaout MA. Polycystin 1 is required for the structural integrity of blood vessels. Proc Natl Acad Sci. 2000;97(4):1731–6. https://doi.org/10.1073/pnas.040550097.

42. Perrone RD, Malek AM, Watnick T. Vascular complications in autosomal dominant polycystic kidney disease. Nat Rev Nephrol. 2015;11(10):589–98. https://doi.org/10.1038/nrneph.2015.128.

43. Lee CH, Ahn C, Ryu H, Kang HS, Jeong SK, Jung KH. Clinical factors associated with the risk of intracranial aneurysm rupture in autosomal dominant polycystic kidney disease. Cerebrovasc Dis. 2021;50(3):339–46. https://doi.org/10.1159/000513709.

44. Kataoka H, Akagawa H, Ushio Y, et al. Mutation type and intracranial aneurysm formation in autosomal dominant polycystic kidney disease. Stroke. 2022;2(5). https://doi.org/10.1161/SVIN.121.000203.

45. Kataoka H, Akagawa H, Yoshida R, et al. Impact of kidney function and kidney volume on intracranial aneurysms in patients with autosomal dominant polycystic kidney disease. Sci Rep. 2022;12(1):18056. https://doi.org/10.1038/s41598-022-22884-9.

46. Flahault A, Joly D. Screening for intracranial aneurysms in patients with autosomal dominant polycystic kidney disease. Clin J Am Soc Nephrol. 2019;14(8):1242–4. https://doi.org/10.2215/CJN.02100219.

47. Scharf E, Pelkowski S, Sahin B. Unruptured intracranial aneurysms and life insurance underwriting. Neurol Clin Pract. 2017;7(3):274–7.

48. Ignacio KHD, Pascual JSG, Factor SJV, et al. A meta-analysis on the prevalence of anxiety and depression in patients with unruptured intracranial aneurysms: exposing critical treatment gaps. Neurosurg Rev. 2022;45:2077–85.

49. van der Schaaf IC, Brilstra EH, Rinkel GJ, Bossuyt PM, van Gijn J. Quality of life, anxiety, and depression in patients with an untreated intracranial aneurysm or arteriovenous malformation. Stroke. 2002;33(2):440–3.

50. Thompson BG, Brown RD Jr, Amin-Hanjani S, Broderick JP, Cockroft KM, Connolly ES Jr, Duckwiler GR, Harris CC, Howard VJ, Johnston SC, Meyers PM, Molyneux A, Ogilvy CS, Ringer AJ, Torner J, American Heart Association Stroke Council, Council on Cardiovascular and Stroke Nursing, and Council on Epidemiology and Prevention, American Heart Association, & American Stroke Association. Guidelines for the management of patients with unruptured intracranial aneurysms: a guideline for healthcare professionals from the American Heart Association/American Stroke Association. Stroke. 2015;46(8):2368–400.

51. Hu S, Yu N, Li Y, Hao Z, Liu Z, Li MH. A meta-analysis of risk factors for the formation of de novo intracranial aneurysms. Neurosurgery. 2019;85(4):454–65.

52. Ogilvy CS, Gomez-Paz S, Kicielinski KP, Salem MM, Akamatsu Y, Waqas M, Rai HH, Catapano JS, Muram S, Elghareeb M, Siddiqui AH, Levy EI, Lawton MT, Mitha AP, Hoh BL, Polifka A, Fox WC, Moore JM, Thomas AJ. Cigarette smoking and risk of intracranial aneurysms in middle-aged women. J Neurol Neurosurg Psychiatry. 2020;91(9):985–90.

53. Huhtakangas J, Numminen J, Pekkola J, Niemelä M, Korja M. Screening of unruptured intracranial aneurysms in 50 to 60-year-old female smokers: a pilot study. Sci Rep. 2021;11(1):23729.

54. Schatlo B, Gautschi OP, Friedrich CM, Ebeling C, Jägersberg M, Kulcsár Z, Pereira VM, Schaller K, Bijlenga P. Association of single and

multiple aneurysms with tobacco abuse: an @neurIST risk analysis. Neurosurg Focus. 2019;47(1):E9.

55. Ogilvy CS, Gomez-Paz S, Kicielinski KP, Salem MM, Maragkos GA, Lee M, Vergara-Garcia D, Rojas R, Moore JM, Thomas AJ. Women with first-hand tobacco smoke exposure have a higher likelihood of having an unruptured intracranial aneurysm than nonsmokers: A nested case-control study. Neurosurgery. 2020;87(6):1191–8.

56. Salih M, Salem MM, Moore JM, Ogilvy CS. Optimal cost-effective screening strategy for unruptured intracranial aneurysms in female smokers. Neurosurgery. 2023;92(1):150–8.

57. Van Hoe W, van Loon J, Demeestere J, Lemmens R, Peluso J, De Vleeschouwer S. Screening for intracranial aneurysms in individuals with a positive first-degree family history: a systematic review. World Neurosurg. 2021;151:235–248.e5.

58. Konovalov A, Grebenev F, Savinkov R, Grebennikov D, Zheltkova V, Bocharov G, Telyshev D, Eliava S. Mathematical analysis of the effectiveness of screening for intracranial aneurysms in first-degree relatives of persons with subarachnoid hemorrhage. World Neurosurg. 2023;175:e542–73.

59. Kim ST, Brinjikji W, Kallmes DF. Prevalence of intracranial aneurysms in patients with connective tissue diseases: a retrospective study. AJNR Am J Neuroradiol. 2016;37(8):1422–6.

60. Gaberel T, Rochey A, di Palma C, Lucas F, Touze E, Emery E. Ruptured intracranial aneurysm in patients with osteogenesis imperfecta: 2 familial cases and a systematic review of the literature. Neurochirurgie. 2016;62(6):317–20.

61. Etminan N, Rinkel GJ. Unruptured intracranial aneurysms: development, rupture and preventive management. Nat Rev Neurol. 2016;12(12):699–713.

62. Perez-Vega C, Domingo RA, Tripathi S, Ramos-Fresnedo A, Martínez Santos JL, Rahme RJ, Freeman WD, Sandhu SS, Miller DA, Bendok BR, Brinjikji W, Quinones-Hinojosa A, Meyer FB, Tawk RG, Fox WC. Intracranial aneurysms in Loeys-Dietz syndrome: a multicenter propensity-matched analysis. Neurosurgery. 2022;91(4):541–6. https://doi.org/10.1227/neu.0000000000002070. Epub 2022 Jul 14. PMID: 35876667

63. Domingo RA, Perez-Vega C, Tripathi S, Santos JM, Ramos-Fresnedo A, Erben YM, Freeman WD, Sandhu SS, Huynh T, Williams L, Bendok BR, Brinjikji W, Tawk RG, Fox WC. Intracranial aneurysms in patients with Marfan syndrome: a multicenter propensity-matched analysis. World Neurosurg. 2021;155:e345–52. https://doi.org/10.1016/j.wneu.2021.08.065. Epub 2021 Aug 21. PMID: 34425290

64. Cheng HC, Faughnan ME, terBrugge KG, Liu HM, Krings T, Brain Vascular Malformation Consortium Hereditary Hemorrhagic Telangiectasia Investigator Group. Prevalence and characteristics of

intracranial aneurysms in hereditary hemorrhagic telangiectasia. AJNR Am J Neuroradiol. 2023;44(12):1367–72.

65. Ring NY, Latif MA, Hafezi-Nejad N, Holly BP, Weiss CR. Prevalence of and factors associated with arterial aneurysms in patients with hereditary hemorrhagic telangiectasia: 17-year retrospective series of 418 patients. J Vasc Interv Radiol. 2021;32(12):1661–9.

66. Abecassis IJ, Xu DS, Batjer HH, Bendok BR. Natural history of brain arteriovenous malformations: a systematic review. Neurosurg Focus. 2014;37(3):E7. https://doi.org/10.3171/2014.6.FOCUS14250. PMID: 25175445

67. Chalouhi N, Hoh BL, Hasan D. Review of cerebral aneurysm formation, growth, and rupture. Stroke. 2013;44(12):3613–22.

68. Newburger JW, Takahashi M, Burns JC. Kawasaki disease. J Am Coll Cardiol.   2016;67(14):1738–49.   https://doi.org/10.1016/j. jacc.2015.12.073.

69. Laukka D, Rahi M, Parkkola R, Vahlberg T, Rintala A, Salo E, Rinne J. Unlikely association between Kawasaki disease and intracranial aneurysms: a prospective cohort study. J Neurosurg Pediatr. 2019:1–4. Advance online publication

70. Laukka D, Kangas E, Kuusela A, et al. Low and borderline ankle-brachial index is associated with intracranial aneurysms: a retrospective cohort   study.   Neurosurgery.   2024;   https://doi.org/10.1227/ neu.0000000000002837.

71. Yan S, Liu Y, Liu C, Yang L, Qin Y, Liu R, Wang S, Li X, Yang W, Ma L, You C, Zhou L, Tian R. Sellar region lesions and intracranial aneurysms in the era of endoscopic endonasal approach. Front Endocrinol. 2021;12:802426.

72. Hobson-Webb LD, Proia AD, Thurberg BL, Banugaria S, Prater SN, Kishnani PS. Autopsy findings in late-onset Pompe disease: a case report and systematic review of the literature. Mol Genet Metab. 2012;106(4):462–9.

73. Vanherpe P, Fieuws S, D'Hondt A, Bleyenheuft C, Demaerel P, De Bleecker J, Van den Bergh P, Baets J, Remiche G, Verhoeven K, Delstanche S, Toussaint M, Buyse B, Van Damme P, Depuydt CE, Claeys KG. Late-onset Pompe disease (LOPD) in Belgium: clinical characteristics and outcome measures. Orphanet J Rare Dis. 2020;15(1):83.

74. Montagnese F, Granata F, Musumeci O, et al. Intracranial arterial abnormalities in patients with late onset Pompe disease (LOPD). J Inherit Metab Dis. 2016;39(3):391–8. https://doi.org/10.1007/s10545-015-9913-x.

75. Musumeci O, Marino S, Granata F, Morabito R, Bonanno L, Brizzi T, Lo Buono V, Corallo F, Longo M, Toscano A. Central nervous system involvement in late-onset Pompe disease: clues from neuroimaging and neuropsychological analysis. Eur J Neurol. 2019;26(3):442–e35.

76. Olin JW, Froehlich J, Gu X, Bacharach JM, Eagle K, Gray BH, Jaff MR, Kim ES, Mace P, Matsumoto AH, McBane RD, Kline-Rogers E, White CJ, Gornik HL. The United States Registry for Fibromuscular Dysplasia: results in the first 447 patients. Circulation. 2012;125(25):3182–90.

77. Slovut DP, Olin JW. Fibromuscular dysplasia. N Engl J Med. 2004;350(18):1862–71.

78. Lather HD, Gornik HL, Olin JW, Gu X, Heidt ST, Kim ESH, Kadian-Dodov D, Sharma A, Gray B, Jaff MR, Chi YW, Mace P, Kline-Rogers E, Froehlich JB. Prevalence of intracranial aneurysm in women with fibromuscular dysplasia: a report from the US registry for fibromuscular dysplasia. JAMA Neurol. 2017;74(9):1081–7.

79. Warchol-Celinska E, Prejbisz A, Dobrowolski P, Klisiewicz A, Kadziela J, Florczak E, Michalowska I, Jozwik-Plebanek K, Kabat M, Kwiatek P, Nazarewski S, Madej K, Rowinski O, Swiatlowski L, Peczkowska M, Hanus K, Talarowska P, Smolski M, Kowalczyk K, Kurkowska-Jastrzebska I, et al. Systematic and multidisciplinary evaluation of fibromuscular dysplasia patients reveals high prevalence of previously undetected fibromuscular dysplasia lesions and affects clinical decisions: the ARCADIA-POL study. Hypertension. 2020;75(4):1102–9.

80. Padilha IG, Guilbert F, Létourneau-Guillon L, Forté S, Nelson K, Bélair M, Raymond J, Soulières D. Should magnetic resonance angiography be used for screening of intracranial aneurysm in adults with sickle cell disease? J Clin Med. 2022;11(24):7463.

81. Stotesbury H, Kawadler JM, Hales PW, Saunders DE, Clark CA, Kirkham FJ. Vascular instability and neurological morbidity in sickle cell disease: An integrative framework. Front Neurol. 2019;10:871.

82. Thust SC, Burke C, Siddiqui A. Neuroimaging findings in sickle cell disease. Br J Radiol. 2014;87(1040):20130699.

83. Rantasalo V, Gunn J, Kiviniemi T, Hirvonen J, Saarenpää I, Kivelev J, Rahi M, Lassila E, Rinne J, Laukka D. Intracranial aneurysm is predicted by abdominal aortic calcification index: a retrospective case-control study. Atherosclerosis. 2021;334:30–8.

84. Wolf D, Ley K. Immunity and inflammation in atherosclerosis. Circ Res. 2019;124(2):315–27.

85. Hurford R, Taveira I, Kuker W, Rothwell PM, Oxford Vascular Study Phenotyped Cohort. Prevalence, predictors and prognosis of incidental intracranial aneurysms in patients with suspected TIA and minor stroke: a population-based study and systematic review. J Neurol Neurosurg Psychiatry. 2021;92(5):542–8.

86. Ortiz AFH, Suriano ES, Eltawil Y, Sekhon M, Gebran A, Garland M, Cuenca NTR, Cadavid T, Almarie B. Prevalence and risk factors of unruptured intracranial aneurysms in ischemic stroke patients – a global meta-analysis. Surg Neurol Int. 2023;14:222.

87. Yan Y, An X, Ren H, Luo B, Han J, Jin S, Liu L, Huang Y. Prevalence and prognosis of acute ischemic stroke coexisting with unruptured intracranial aneurysms. Front Neurol. 2023;14:1286193.
88. Egbe AC, Padang R, Brown RD, Khan AR, Luis SA, Huston J 3rd, Akintoye E, Connolly HM. Prevalence and predictors of intracranial aneurysms in patients with bicuspid aortic valve. Heart. 2017;103(19):1508–14.
89. Yu X, Xia L, Jiang Q, Wei Y, Wei X, Cao S. Prevalence of intracranial aneurysm in patients with aortopathy: a systematic review with meta-analyses. J Stroke. 2020;22(1):76–86.
90. Vallabhajosyula S, Yang LT, Thomas SC, Maleszewski JJ, Boler AN, Thapa P, Enriquez-Sarano M, Rabinstein AA, Michelena HI. Prevalence and outcomes of bicuspid aortic valve in patients with aneurysmal subarachnoid hemorrhage: a prospective neurology registry report. J Am Heart Assoc. 2022;11(8):e022339.
91. Chen J, Han M, Feng X, Peng F, Tong X, Niu H, Zhang D, Liu A. Cost effectiveness of screening for intracranial aneurysms among patients with bicuspid aortic valve: a Markov modelling study. BMJ Open. 2021;11(12):e051236.
92. Lee D, Ahn SJ, Cho ES, Kim YB, Song SW, Jung WS, Suh SH. High prevalence of intracranial aneurysms in patients with aortic dissection or aneurysm: feasibility of extended aorta CT angiography with involvement of intracranial arteries. J Neurointerv Surg. 2017;9(10):1017–21.
93. Song J, Lim YC, Ko I, Kim JY, Kim DK. Prevalence of intracranial aneurysm in patients with aortic disease in Korea: a Nationwide Population-Based Study. J Am Heart Assoc. 2021;10(6):e019009.
94. Jung WS, Kim JH, Ahn SJ, Song SW, Kim BM, Seo KD, Suh SH. Prevalence of intracranial aneurysms in patients with aortic dissection. AJNR Am J Neuroradiol. 2017;38(11):2089–93.
95. Rouchaud A, Brandt MD, Rydberg AM, Kadirvel R, Flemming K, Kallmes DF, Brinjikji W. Prevalence of intracranial aneurysms in patients with aortic aneurysms. AJNR Am J Neuroradiol. 2016;37(9):1664–8.
96. Song J, Lim YC, Ko I, Kim JY, Kim DK. Prevalence of intracranial aneurysms in patients with systemic vessel aneurysms: a nationwide cohort study. Stroke. 2020;51(1):115–20.
97. Hill HL, Stanley JC, Matusko N, Ganesh SK, Coleman DM. The association of intracranial aneurysms in women with renal artery aneurysms. Ann Vasc Surg. 2019;60:147–155.e2.
98. Prasad M, Tweet MS, Hayes SN, Leng S, Liang JJ, Eleid MF, Gulati R, Vrtiska TJ. Prevalence of extracoronary vascular abnormalities and fibromuscular dysplasia in patients with spontaneous coronary artery dissection. Am J Cardiol. 2015;115(12):1672–7.

99. Li Q, Yang Y, Pan Y, Duan L, Yang H. The quality assessment of clinical practice guidelines for intracranial aneurysms: a systematic appraisal. Neurosurg Rev. 2018;41(2):629–39.

100. Alwalid O, Long X, Xie M, Han P. Artificial intelligence applications in intracranial aneurysm: achievements, challenges and opportunities. Acad Radiol. 2022;29(Suppl 3):S201–14.

101. Heo J, Park SJ, Kang SH, Oh CW, Bang JS, Kim T. Prediction of intracranial aneurysm risk using machine learning. Sci Rep. 2020;10(1):6921.

102. Fiani B, Pasko KBD, Sarhadi K, Covarrubias C. Current uses, emerging applications, and clinical integration of artificial intelligence in neuroradiology. Rev Neurosci. 2021;33(4):383–95.

103. Yu Y, Chen DYT. Machine learning for cerebrovascular disorders. In: Colliot O, editor. Machine learning for brain disorders. New York: Humana; 2023. p. 921–61.

104. Mouridsen K, Thurner P, Zaharchuk G. Artificial intelligence applications in stroke. Stroke. 2020;51(8):2573–9.

105. Qiu T, Jin G, Bao W. The interrelated effects of 2D angiographic morphological variables and aneurysm rupture. Neurosciences. 2014;19(3):210–7.

106. Lau Q, Hsu W, Lee M, Mao Y, Chen L. Prediction of cerebral aneurysm rupture. 2007; 350–357. https://doi.org/10.1109/ICTAI.2007.98.
Kim HC, Rhim JK, Ahn JH, et al. Machine Learning Application for Rupture Risk Assessment in Small-Sized Intracranial Aneurysm. J Clin Med. 2019;8(5):683. Published 2019 May 15. https://doi.org/10.3390/jcm8050683

107. Zhu W, Li W, Tian Z, Zhang Y, Wang K, Zhang Y, et al. Stability assessment of intracranial aneurysms using machine learning based on clinical and morphological features. Transl Stroke Res. 2020;11(6):1287–95.

108. Mocco J, Brown RD Jr, Torner JC, Capuano AW, Fargen KM, Raghavan ML, Piepgras DG, Meissner I, Huston J III, International Study of Unruptured Intracranial Aneurysms Investigators. Aneurysm morphology and prediction of rupture: an International Study of Unruptured Intracranial Aneurysms Analysis. Neurosurgery. 2018;82(4):491–6. https://doi.org/10.1093/neuros/nyx226. PMID: 28605486; PMCID: PMC6256940

109. Vitošević F, Milošević Medenica S, Kalousek V, Mandić-Rajčević S, Vitošević M, Lepić M, Rotim K, Rasulić L. Clinical characteristics and morphological parameters associated with rupture of anterior communicating artery aneurysms. Acta Clin Croat. 2022;61(2):284–94. https://doi.org/10.20471/acc.2022.61.02.15. PMID: 36818935; PMCID: PMC9934047

110. Dhar S, Tremmel M, Mocco J, et al. Morphology parameters for intracranial aneurysm rupture risk assessment. Neurosurgery. 2008;63(2):185–97. https://doi.org/10.1227/01.NEU.0000316847.64140.81.

111. Shi Z, Chen GZ, Mao L, Li XL, Zhou CS, Xia S, et al. Machine learning-based prediction of small intracranial aneurysm rupture status using CTA-derived hemodynamics: a multicenter study. AJNR Am J Neuroradiol. 2021;42(4):648–54.

112. Tanioka S, Ishida F, Yamamoto A, Shimizu S, Sakaida H, Toyoda M, et al. Machine learning classification of cerebral aneurysm rupture status with morphologic variables and hemodynamic parameters. Radiol Artif Intell. 2020;2(1):e190077.

113. Chen R, Mo X, Chen Z, Feng P, Li H. An integrated model combining machine learning and deep learning algorithms for classification of rupture status of IAs. Front Neurol. 2022;13:868395.

Endovascular Management and Treatment of Acute Ischemic Stroke

10

Omer Doron, Yafell Serulle,
Likowsky L. Desir, Hamza Khilji,
and Rafael Ortiz

Introduction

Stroke is a leading cause of disability and death in the modern society [1]. Aging population, modern lifestyle, and other contributing factors such as ischemic heart disease, atherosclerosis, unbalanced diet, smoking, and hypertension are among known risk factors [2]. While a steady improvement in recognizing and modifying prevention strategies to battle the epidemic of ischemic stroke has taken place over last few decades, the past decade has seen a giant leap in the development and implementation of ischemic stroke treatment, in particular large vessel occlusion type [3].

Multiple technological advancements have evolved simultaneously, contributing to a revolution in the field. Starting at the prehospital phase where awareness and population's education became more prevalent, going through advanced imaging tools

O. Doron · Y. Serulle · L. L. Desir · H. Khilji · R. Ortiz (✉)
Department of Neurosurgery, Lenox Hill Hospital, Donald and Barbara
Zucker School of Medicine at Hofstra/Northwell Health,
New York, NY, USA
e-mail: Rortiz3@northwell.edu

© The Author(s), under exclusive license to Springer Nature
Switzerland AG 2025
E. Veznedaroglu (ed.), *Advanced Technologies in Vascular
Neurosurgery*, https://doi.org/10.1007/978-3-031-67492-1_10

allowing for a quick and accurate triage and decision-making, culminating in the cerebral angiography suit where new techniques and devices were created to allow quick clot aspiration and an effective removal, realizing the notion that "time is brain" [4, 5].

As the science of stroke care is still developing, this chapter will survey major advancements made in the past 20 years in the field of ischemic stroke treatment, as it was, and still is, being transformed. While successful studies are recognized and their conclusions will be brought forward and discussed, we also sought to describe trials that failed during this time span, as often failed devices or treatment strategies that were abandoned served as fuel for more innovative approaches, after understanding the reasons for specific failures.

The revolution of acute ischemic stroke treatment in many ways pushed the relatively new field of endovascular neurosurgery, which was heavily dominated by aneurysm treatment. Thus, innovations in imaging techniques—understanding how to locate and accurately assess salvageable brain tissue—and innovations in catheter-based intervention techniques are the two main drivers and prisms through which we describe the newly formed paradigms in this chapter.

Importantly, new technologies bring new therapeutic opportunities as well as controversies which are brought in the last part of this chapter, as we discuss alternative triage modalities, such as direct angio-suite, artificial intelligence-driven image processing which governs present software market, neuroprotection strategies which may facilitate longer treatment windows, and devices and techniques for middle-sized vessel occlusions (MVOs).

The Introduction of Intravenous and Intra-arterial rtPA: The Pre-thrombectomy Era

Large vessel occlusions (LVOs) typically refer to acute blockages found in the larger intracranial vessels: internal carotid artery (ICA), proximal middle cerebral artery (MCA), and basilar artery. Given that LVOs are responsible for 46% of the acute ischemic strokes (AISs) suffered by 700,000 individuals in the USA, annually, and have twice the risk of death or dependence when compared to non-LVO AISs from the pre-endovascular area, their clinical relevance is significant [6–8].

Before modern treatments, the AIS early mortality rate was 10% [9]. Among survivors, approximately half presented with moderate-to-severe neurologic deficits, and a quarter were dependent on others. AIS data from a meta-analysis preceding the endovascular era and observational data from mixed populations of AIS patients (many presenting outside of the tPA window) both demonstrated that rates of dependence or death at 3 to 6 months (defined by a modified Rankin scale (mRS) score of 3–6) were more than double for patients with LVO versus non-LVOs (64 vs. 24%, $P < 0.0001$). Additionally, the 6-month mortality rates were also significantly higher in AIS patients with LVO versus without LVO (26.2 vs. 1.3%, $P < 0.0001$) [10].

Even among patients with TIAs or minor strokes (defined as ≤3 on the 42-point National Institutes of Health Stroke Scale (NIHSS)), LVO presence correlated with a significant increase in the rate of recurrent stroke (45.8 vs. 5.8%, $P < 0.001$) and functional impairment (37.5 vs. 7.7) within 90 days [11]. This likely resulted from embolic events distal to the LVO and/or inadequacy of collateral perfusion over time. Moreover, the stroke severity and overall clinical outcomes in AIS patients (as defined by the NIHSS score) were impacted by the occlusion location and number of occluded vessels [9].

The introduction of intravenous alteplase in 1995 led to substantial improvement in AIS outcomes [12]. The first effective treatment for acute stroke originated from a randomized controlled trial that resulted in the approval of intravenously administered recombinant tissue-type plasminogen activator (r-tPA). This randomized, double-blind trial of intravenous recombinant tissue plasminogen activator (t-PA) for ischemic stroke was conducted after recent pilot studies had suggested the benefit of t-PA when used as a treatment within 3 hours of the onset of a stroke [13].

Patient eligibility for this two-part trial was contingent upon a history of an ischemic stroke with a clearly defined time of onset, a deficit measurable on the NIHSS, and a baseline computed tomographic (CT) scan of the brain that showed no evidence of intracranial hemorrhage. The first part, consisting of 291 patients, tested the clinical activity of t-PA, which was defined as an improvement of 4 points over baseline values in the score of the NIHSS scale or the resolution of the neurologic deficit within 24 hours of the stroke onset. Between the group given t-PA and that given placebo, the results demonstrated no significant difference in the percentages of patients with neurologic improvement at 24 hours, although a benefit was observed for the t-PA group at 3 months for all four outcome measures [14, 15].

In the second part, consisting of 333 enrolled patients, the clinical outcome at 3 months, according to scores on the Barthel index, modified Rankin scale, Glasgow outcome scale, and NIHSS, was assessed.

The long-term clinical benefit of t-PA predicted by the results from part one of the trial was confirmed (global odds ratio for a favorable outcome, 1.7 [1.2–1.6, CI 95%]). When compared with patients given a placebo, patients treated with t-PA were at least 30% more likely to have minimal or no disability at 3 months on the assessment scales. In a later meta-analysis of nine randomized controlled trials assessing the impact of intravenous alteplase [16], 32.9% of the patients in the alteplase group, as compared with 23.1% of the patients in the control group, had a favorable 3-month outcome (defined as a mRS 0–1) when treatment was administered within 3 hours after the onset of stroke (adjusted odds ratio 1.75 [1.35–2.27, CI 95%]); the corresponding rates were 35.3% and 30.1% when treatment was administered between 3 and 4.5 hours after onset (adjusted odds ratio, 1.26 [1.05–1.51, CI 95%]). Large intracerebral hemorrhage occurred in 6.8% of the patients in the alteplase group and in 1.3% of those in the control group.

The benefits of r-tPA were further underscored by multiple additional studies and pooled analyses over the next two decades [17–19]. As a result, in 1995, the administration of tPA became the standard of care for AIS patients presenting within 3 hours of symptom onset. In 2008, this timeframe was extended to 4.5 hours [17].

Despite its status as a breakthrough in management of AIS patients, the benefits of IV rtPA therapy were still somewhat limited in patients with LVO [20]. This stemmed from the fact that LVOs were commonly refractory to tPA, with resistance to pharmacologic thrombolysis increasing with more proximal occlusions (31–44% recanalization rate with tPA for M2 occlusions vs. 4–8% for ICA terminus LVOs) [21–23]. As a result, r-tPA provided an incomplete benefit to patients needing it the most: those who suffered severe strokes which rendered them severely disabled or dead. This promoted interest in intra-arterial therapies in which large artery clots would lyse more effectively.

The PROACT trials, which were conducted between 1996 and 1999, introduced the initial push for intra-arterial treatment for ischemic stroke [24, 25]. In these studies, radiological assessment played a critical role in determining patient eligibility, as patients were excluded on the basis of hemorrhage and any subtle signs showing low likelihood of recovery after irreversible cerebral parenchymatic changes, such as acute hypodense parenchymal lesion or effacement of cerebral sulci in more than one third of the MCA territory (taken from European Cooperative Acute Stroke Study [ECASS] criteria).

Furthermore, once enrolled, diagnostic cerebral angiography of the symptomatic MCA territory documentation and specific findings, such as complete occlusion or minimal perfusion of either the M_1 segment or an M_2 division of the MCA, were required. Additional exclusion criteria included pathologies such as arterial dissection, severe arterial stenosis precluding safe passage of a microcatheter into the MCA, non-atherosclerotic arteriopathy, no visible occlusion, or occlusion of an artery other than the M_1 or M_2 division of the MCA. Hence, this was one of the first large trials weeding out stroke patients based on likelihood of response to therapy predicated on imaging.

In the PROACT trials, an infusion microcatheter (<3.0 F) with a single end hole was placed into the proximal one third of the MCA thrombus. If intrathrombus positioning of the infusion catheter was not possible, the tip of the catheter was placed as close to the proximal face of the thrombus as possible for r-proUK infusion.

A superselective angiogram was performed through the micro-catheter to document catheter placement, and mechanical disruption of the clot was not permitted. Recombinant prourokinase was then infused, and another angiogram was performed through the microcatheter.

If any of the proximal thrombus had dissolved, the operator advanced the microcatheter tip into the proximal portion of any remaining clot in the MCA. Finally, a diagnostic carotid angiogram was performed at 2 hours to assess vessel patency.

PROACT I demonstrated that IAT administration of 6 mg prourokinase in patients with M1 or M2 occlusions resulted in higher recanalization rates relative to standard therapy.

In PROACT II, patients with angiographically proven proximal MCA occlusions were randomized to receive IAT with 9 mg of prourokinase (given proximal to the clot and mechanical clot disruption with the guidewire was not allowed) plus heparin, or heparin only in the control arm.

Prourokinase administration within 6 hours resulted in a significantly higher number of patients with a mRS score of 2 or less at 90 days (40% vs. 25%), with recanalization rates of 66% vs. 18%. However, symptomatic intracranial hemorrhage occurred in 10% versus 2% in controls, and mortality was 25% versus 27% in controls.

Mechanical Thrombectomy: The Early Years and Failed Trials

Advancements in the field of neuroendovascular intervention led to the development of the MERCI Retriever. This device included a flexible nickel titanium (nitinol) wire that formed a helical shape once it was passed through the tip of the guidance catheter (Fig. 10.1).

In practice, the catheter/wire was passed distal to the thrombus, and then removed, with the wire assuming helical configuration. The clot was then trapped in the helix and withdrawn from the vasculature. This helically coiled tip device, designed to grasp the clot for removal, previously had marketing authorization for retrieval of foreign bodies misplaced during interventional

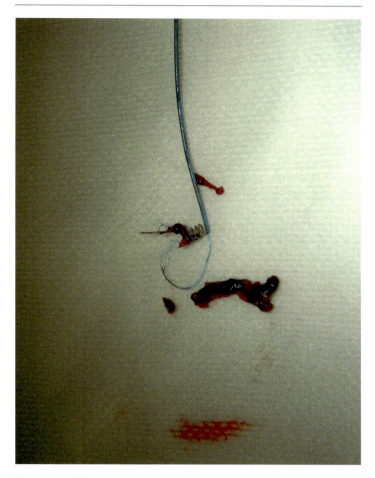

Fig. 10.1   MERCI device used in this case to retrieve a clot from the cerebral vasculature in the early days of mechanical thrombectomy

radiological procedures in the peripheral and coronary vascular systems.

The MERCI trial was a prospective, single-arm, multicenter trial conducted at 25 US centers [26]. The study tested whether a mechanical embolectomy device, when utilized by a trained interventional neuroradiologist, could safely restore vascular patency at a rate exceeding a prespecified rate of spontaneous recanalization in patients presenting within 8 hours of onset of an AIS. Additionally, the device design, performance, and the adequacy of the instructions for use were evaluated. The trial was designed to assess the least burdensome method of obtaining safety and efficacy data that could lead to FDA clearance of the tool with a specific indication of mechanical thrombectomy in the neurovasculature [27].

The radiographic inclusion criteria were similar to the ones used for the PROACT II trial. Stroke symptom duration was required to be between 3 and 8 hours, or duration between 0 and 3 hours, and a contraindication for intravenous tPA. Intra-arterial thrombolytics were allowed in cases of treatment failure with the device or to treat distal embolus not accessible to the device after successful proximal embolectomy.

The neurological outcome, which should be the most important outcome in a stroke treatment trial, was a secondary end point in the MERCI study and was again determined by comparing the outcome of treated patients to the placebo arm of PROACT II. Similar to PROACT II, MERCI included patients with M1 and M2 occlusions but also included patients with occlusions of the supraclinoid internal carotid artery (9%) and the vertebral basilar system (14%), making direct comparisons of outcomes difficult, as these are associated with high mortality if the vessel fails to open with intra-arterial thrombolytic therapy.

The results showed successful revascularization in 46% of patients on intention-to-treat analysis and in 48% of patients who were treated with the device. This was significantly greater than the 18% spontaneous recanalization rate of the middle cerebral artery reported in the PROACT II study, confirming that the device could efficiently restore blood flow.

Despite the efficacy of the device, the MERCI trial had several limitations. The overall mortality in the MERCI trial was 44%, greater than most prospective trials of acute stroke at the time. The 45% recanalization of the MCA in the MERCI trial was less than the 66% rate reported with intra-arterial prourokinase.

Importantly, the MERCI symptomatic intracranial hemorrhage rate was best estimated at 7 of 141 (5%), higher than the rates of intracranial hemorrhage in the placebo arms of the NINDS intravenous tPA trial (0.6%) and the placebo arm of the intra-arterial prourokinase trial PROACT-II (2%) but less than the rates of hemorrhage from intravenous tPA (6% in NINDS study), combined intravenous/intra-arterial tPA (6% in the IMS trial [28]), or intra-arterial prourokinase (10% in PROACT-II). Therefore, the symptomatic intracranial bleeding rates were in fact smaller than those from existing treatments for acute ischemic stroke.

Based on the MERCI trial results, the FDA cleared the MERCI Retriever in 2004 for restoring blood flow in patients experiencing an acute stroke who were otherwise ineligible for intravenous tPA or in whom intravenous tPA treatment was unsuccessful.

The MULTI MERCI trial, an international trial which included a newer generation (L5 model) of the MERCI device and patients who had failed IV tPA, demonstrated that mechanical thrombectomy after IV tPA was as safe as mechanical thrombectomy alone [26].

This first generation of mechanical thrombectomy devices was approved by the FDA and propelled an era of interventional stroke trials. In addition, sub-analysis showed that patients with successful recanalization were more likely to achieve good clinical outcome, thereby establishing a clinical rationale for early recanalization after acute stroke that subsequently fueled the pursuit after more efficacious methods.

In order to improve mechanical thrombectomy success rate, an aspiration system, preceding clot retrieval attempts, was introduced. The Penumbra aspiration System (PS) was tested in the Penumbra Pivotal Stroke Trial, published in 2009 [29].

This trial was a nonrandomized, prospective, single-arm, 125-patient study designed to assess the safety and effectiveness of the PS in reducing clot burden in acute ischemic stroke using the MERCI clot retriever (Concentric Medical) as the predicate device and historical control.

The goal of the trial was to support "substantial equivalence" in safety and effectiveness of the system to the MERCI device in opening clotted cerebral blood vessels in stroke.

The PS was specifically designed to provide two revascularization options: thrombus debulking and aspiration, followed by direct thrombus extraction if clots remained. This was attained by appropriate catheter position proximal to the clot, as the penumbra separator was advanced through the penumbra reperfusion catheter. The penumbra aspiration pump was then turned on to initiate revascularization. Reduction of the clot burden by aspiration was accomplished by connecting the reperfusion catheter to the penumbra aspiration pump, which generated a vacuum of 20 inches/Hg.

A continuous aspiration-debulking process was facilitated by advancing and withdrawing the separator through the Penumbra reperfusion catheter into the proximal end of the clot. If the thrombus remained, a second accessory method of direct mechanical retrieval by the thrombus removal ring was used to enhance revascularization. Thrombus extraction using the thrombus removal ring was accomplished by engaging the clot proximally and extracting the clot under flow arrest conditions by inflating a proximal balloon guide catheter. This technique, in many ways, is the basis for present mechanical thrombectomy.

The results showed that, postprocedure, 81.6% of the treated vessels were successfully revascularized to TICI 2 to 3. The rate of serious procedural adverse events was 2.4% and 11.2% in the patients who suffered symptomatic ICH. All-cause mortality was 32.8% at 90 days with 25% of the patients achieving a mRS score of 2. Overall, the PS showed substantial safety and efficacy and was cleared for clinical use.

As for the clinical outcome regarding AIS treatment, the authors stated that "heterogeneous study population may be a contributing factor because imaging was not used to define the presence of salvageable ischemic penumbra at study entry. The absence of imaging-guided patient selection and a historical control design may render elusive a definitive conclusion on long-term outcome." The path for studying the actual effect of revascularization on clinical outcome was therefore not resolved without a controlled trial using clearly defined tools for imaging-guided patient selection, an assertation which would prove to be crucial later on.

Mechanical thrombectomy devices continued to evolve with the appearance of the stent retrievers, or stentrievers, which are self-expandable stents for thrombectomy designed to be deployed at the site of the occlusion.

Deploying the stent retriever involves first crossing the occlusion with a microcatheter typically over a microwire. Once distal to the occlusion, the stent retriever is then expanded to capture the thrombus, which immediately may restore blood flow. Theoretically, such flow restoration would enhance the efficacy of systemic thrombolytic drugs if already in the circulation.

After a period of usually 3–5 minutes depending of the location and clot size, the stent can be retrieved by pulling it back into the guide catheter under proximal aspiration. Some techniques have advocated the addition of a proximal balloon guide catheter (BGC) could aid aspiration and help thrombus retrieval when the stent retriever is being dragged back into the guide catheter, preventing distal embolization of captured clots during clot retrieval through the arrest of blood flow [30].

The first stent retriever developed was Solitaire (Medtronic Neurovascular, Irvine, CA, USA), which was approved by FDA in 2012 and quickly became the first choice for many practitioners following the success of the Solitaire with the Intention for Thrombectomy (SWIFT) trial [31].

This randomized, parallel-group, noninferiority trial consisted of enrolled patients from 18 sites who were allocated for thrombectomy treatment with either Solitaire or MERCI. Successful recanalization of TICI grade 2 or 3 was achieved in 60.7% of patients in the Solitaire group but only 24.1% in the MERCI group. The clinical outcome, defined by a mRS 0 to 2 at 3 months (58.2% vs. 33.6%) and mortality (17.2% vs. 38.2%), was favorable for the Solitaire stent as well, solidifying the efficacy of mechanical thrombectomy devices.

The TREVO embolectomy device was introduced shortly afterward (Stryker Neurovascular, Fremont, CA, USA). It was an alternative stent retriever device that could be advanced through a microcatheter past the occlusion site and deployed to cover the entire thrombus in a manner similar to the technique of Solitaire. The TREVO retriever has various lineups, with one distinguishing

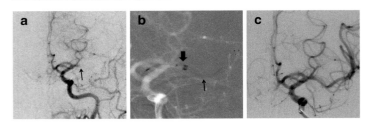

Fig. 10.2 Patient with a left middle cerebral artery occlusion undergoing mechanical thrombectomy. (**a**) Injection of the left internal carotid artery demonstrates total occlusion of the proximal M1 segment of the left middle cerebral artery (the arrow demonstrates the site of the occlusion). (**b**) Endovascular mechanical thrombectomy is performed by advancing an aspiration catheter into the left middle cerebral artery just proximal to the clot (thick arrow). A stent retriever is then deployed through a microcatheter across the area of the clot (thin arrow). (**c**) Following aspiration and retrieval of the stent retriever, injection of the left internal carotid artery demonstrates complete recanalization of the vessel

feature of this retriever being fully visible stent strut under fluoroscopy (Fig. 10.2).

The Thrombectomy Revascularization of Large Vessel Occlusions in Acute Ischemic Stroke (TREVO 2) trial [32] demonstrated the success of the TREVO device in comparison to the MERCI device in a similar fashion to the SWIFT trial. Recanalization rates with a Thrombolysis in Cerebral Ischemia (TICI) 2 or 3 were 86% in the TREVO group versus 60% in the MERCI group, but there was no statistically significant difference regarding procedure-related adverse events between the two groups (15% in the TREVO group vs. 23% in the MERCI group, $p = 0.18$).

Comparing SWIFT and TREVO 2 trials was not straightforward. The primary end point in the SWIFT trial was thrombolysis in myocardial ischemia scale 2 or 3 and flow in all treatable vessels without symptomatic intracranial hemorrhage after ≤3 passes of the assigned device, assessed by an independent core laboratory that was masked to study assignment.

The primary end point in the TREVO 2 trial was a thrombolysis in cerebral infarction scale 2 or 3 and flow with the assigned device alone, evaluated by an unmasked central imaging core.

The use of different scoring scales, differences in masking of study assignment, and lack of information on reperfusion by location of vessel occlusion complicate comparison between reperfusion rates for the two stent retrievers.

Safety is where the two trials differed. The SWIFT trial reported a lower 90-day mortality rate in the Solitaire group than the MERCI group (17% vs. 38%; OR, 0.34 [0.14–0.81]) and lower rates of symptomatic intracerebral hemorrhage (ICH; Solitaire 2% vs. MERCI 11%; OR, 0.14 [0.02–1.23]). In the TREVO 2 trial, the 90-day mortality rates (stent retriever 33% vs. MERCI 24%; OR, 1.61 [0.83–3.13]) and symptomatic ICH rates (stent retriever 7% vs. MERCI 9%; OR, 0.75 [0.25–2.26]) were not significantly different. Symptomatic ICH in both trials used the European Cooperative Acute Stroke Study III criteria [33].

The higher rates of mortality and symptomatic ICH in the MERCI group compared with the Solitaire group in the SWIFT trial are likely due to improved reperfusion with the stent retriever and differences in the rates of IV tPA between the treatment arms and particularly the use of additional mechanical thrombectomy devices in the MERCI group and in the SWIFT trial (44% of the MERCI group had additional endovascular treatment with various mechanical devices used after the MERCI Retriever, which may have led to additional complications).

In contrast, the MERCI group in the TREVO II trial depicted a trend toward a lower 90-day mortality rate compared with the stent retriever group, despite much better overall outcomes with regard to mRS of 0 to 2 in the stent retriever group. These variances in mortality between the trials highlight the limitations of smaller randomized trials, in which more extreme discrepancies between groups can be observed due to imbalances in important prognostic variables, other treatments, or simply chance. Both of these trials indicate that the stent retriever devices are preferable to the MERCI Retriever when endovascular therapy is considered.

In March 2013, three randomized controlled trials, SYNTHESIS, MR RESCUE, and IMS III [34, 35], were presented at the International Stroke Conference in Hawaii and subsequently published in the same issue of the *New England Journal of Medicine*. However, all three trials reported negative results.

The SYNTHESIS trial compared endovascular therapy, in the form of intra-arterial thrombolysis with rtPA, mechanical clot disruption or retrieval, or a combination of these approaches, to treatment with IV tPA alone. Demonstration of vessel occlusion prior to endovascular treatment was not required nor was any clinical severity rating on the NIHSS, and the reperfusion rates were not reported. There was no difference in good clinical outcome, with 42% in the endovascular arm versus 46% in the intravenous tPA arm. A mechanical device was only used in 56 out of 181 patients randomized to endovascular treatment; however, this trial did implement the use of retrievable stents, the third generation of mechanical devices, in 23 out of 56 patients in whom a device was deployed.

IMS III was a large, randomized controlled trial comparing endovascular therapy plus IVT (IVT stopped at 40 min) to IVT alone. Demonstration of intracranial occlusion was not required. In IMS III, an NIHSS ≥ 10 was used as a marker of stroke severity and risk of proximal occlusion, but as computed tomography angiography (CTA) was popularized, an amendment midway through the trial allowed screening for proximal clots with CTA for patients with NIHSS of 8 or 9. No Penumbra assessment was carried out in this trial, and it was similar to previous trials in terms of reliance on CT findings. More advanced therapies were allowed, including MERCI, Penumbra, Solitaire, or Microcatheter delivery of intra-arterial tPA. As a result, the methods were a mix of pharmacological thrombolysis, manipulation of clot using a guidewire or microcatheter, mechanical and aspiration thrombectomy, and stent retriever technology. The procedure was required to begin within 5 hours.

The results demonstrated that there was no difference in outcome between groups, with 41% good clinical outcome (mRS 0–2) in the combined IVT/EVT arm versus 39% in the IVT-only arm. Recanalization rate (defined as modified arterial occlusion lesion score mAOL 2–3) was 81% for ICA occlusion and 86% for M1 occlusion; the reperfusion rate (mTICI 2b/3) was 38% for ICA occlusion and 44% for M1 occlusion. The retrievable stents were only used in 14 patients.

The third trial, MR RESCUE, had a duration of 8 years, in which it compared patients receiving endovascular therapy to those receiving standard care via the MERCI Retriever or Penumbra system.

Moreover, it was a unique study since it introduced the concept of penumbral pattern in the pretreatment assessment process in an attempt to stratify patients by incorporating advanced imaging—a key tool that would prove useful in later years. All patients underwent a pretreatment CT or MRI of the brain. Randomization was stratified depending on whether the patient had a favorable penumbral pattern (substantial salvageable tissue and small infarct core) or a nonpenumbral pattern (large core or small or absent penumbra). A favorable penumbral pattern was defined as a predicted infarct core of 90 ml or less and a proportion of predicted infarct tissue within the at-risk region of 70% or less.

Overall, these three trials failed to show a true benefit for endovascular intervention in ischemic stroke. Expectedly, a variety of limitations were identified in all three studies. Firstly, the use of noninvasive angiography was not universal in patient selection. For example, in IMS III, more than 50% of patients did not undergo CTA, as it was not in widespread use during early patient recruitment. In MR RESCUE, patients were eligible only if angiography showed persistent target occlusion after receiving tPA. Secondly, there were long time delays from stroke onset to revascularization, in part due to lack of rapid workflow. Lastly, the devices were relatively limited in their ability to achieve recanalization, and the new generation retrievable stents were used in a small number of patients.

Identification of these flaws has impacted the design of future endovascular therapy RCTs, propelling the incorporation of more uniform, newer-generation device use along with advanced imaging criteria.

Image-Guided Stroke Therapy: The True Impact of Mechanical Thrombectomy

The Impact of Newer-Generation Devices and Uniform Inclusion Criteria

After the 2013 trials, which disrupted the adoption of mechanical thrombectomy as the future of AIS therapy, the first landmark positive trial was MR CLEAN, presented at the ninth World Stroke

Congress in October 2014 [36]. The eligibility for patients was onset within 6 hours, proximal occlusion of the anterior circulation (distal ICA, M1 or M2, first or second portion of anterior cerebral artery, A1 or A2), and an NIHSS score > 2. As a single-country trial conducted in the Netherlands, patients were randomly assigned to either intra-arterial treatment plus usual care or usual care alone.

The uniqueness of this trial stemmed from multiple factors, including the use of baseline vessel imaging (CTA, MRA, or DSA) for the location of the occlusion as an inclusion criteria. Additionally, the vast majority of patients received IVT (89%), and 82% of patients were treated with stent retrievers. Another unique factor was the use of adjusted common odds ratio for a shift in the direction of a better outcome on the mRS rather than a dichotomized mRS as the primary outcome.

The study showed the adjusted common odds ratio was 1.67 (95% CI 1.21–2.30), for patients treated by intra-arterial therapy, representing the first positive RCT for endovascular therapy. More patients achieved functional independence (mRS 0–2) at 90 days in the intervention group, 33% compared to 19% (95% CI 5.9–21.2) with an adjusted odds ratio of 2.16 (95% CI 1.39–3.38), a statistically significant result.

Unlike the IMS III trial and the SYNTHESIS Expansion trial, MR CLEAN required a radiologically proven intracranial occlusion for study eligibility. When the IMS III trial was designed, the availability of CTA was still limited, and the presence of a proximal arterial occlusion was therefore uncertain in a subgroup of patients in that trial (47% of the study population). Thus, a group of patients in which it is likely that intra-arterial treatment would not alter the natural history of acute ischemic stroke was excluded. Moreover, the study benefited from the widespread availability of retrievable stents, which were shown to be superior to the first-generation MERCI device for both revascularization and clinical outcomes. Given that these were used in 82% of the patients in the intervention group, this served as an attestation for the impact of a new technology which was not previously assessed as the major thrombectomy modality.

The ESCAPE trial [37], conducted from February 2013 to October 2014 across 22 sites in Canada, the USA, Ireland, and South Korea, allowed recruitment of patients within 12 hours, the longest time window of all the trials, with clinical severity requirements for inclusion set at an NIHSS >6. Additionally, advanced imaging criteria were required: NCCT ASPECTS >5 aimed at identifying small core infarcts; proximal intracranial occlusion of M1, M2, or intracranial ICA was required on vascular imaging, with tandem occlusion of the extra-cranial internal carotid artery; and moderate to good collaterals, defined as filling of >50% of MCA pial arterial circulation on CTA, preferably acquired with multiphase CTA (being less vulnerable to patient motion than CT perfusion, requires no additional contrast, and allows for quick determination of collateral status). If CT perfusion was used, a low CBV or very low CBF and ASPECTS >5 was needed.

This trial also required an imaging-to-groin puncture time of <60 minutes and a target groin puncture to reperfusion time of <30 minutes. Rapid workflow was emphasized, thus achieving the shortest onset-to-reperfusion time among the trials—the median stroke onset to reperfusion was 4 hours. Of patients, 76% received IVT.

The trial indicated an increase in functional independence (mRS 0–2) at 90 days from 29% in the control group to 53% in the intervention group ($p < 0.001$), and the primary outcome favored the intervention with a common odds ratio of 2.6 (95% CI 1.7–3.8; $p < 0.001$). This trial was the only trial to demonstrate a statistically significant reduction in mortality from 19% to 10% ($p = 0.04$).

As improvement in tools available for neurointerventionalists, as well as speedy intervention, has seemed to propel better outcome, the implementation of the penumbra mapping into the stroke trials was a pertinent, paradigm-shifting concept.

Advanced Imaging and Its Incorporation to the New Stroke Trials

Animal studies have played a major role in understanding the evolution of brain tissue following ischemia. In 1974, Symon et al. [38] demonstrated, in a middle cerebral artery occlusion (MCAo) model of focal stroke in baboons, the presence of large variations in the reduction of cerebral blood flow in ischemic tissue. This signified that the blood flow supplying brain tissue varied depending on the vessel route, indicating that a poststroke treatment was possible by salvaging the tissue at risk of infarction.

In 1977, Astrup et al. [39] utilized the same model to demonstrate that failure of electrical activity was not uniform across an ischemic region, indicating that some tissue remained electrically active despite severe ischemia. Ischemic thresholds were established based on CBF levels.

They identified three regions: below 20 ml/100 g/min, where electrical function of the tissue is affected; below 15 mlv 100 g/min, where electrical failure is complete; and below 5 mlv100 g/min, where release of extracellular K ions attests to impending cell death. Furthermore, it was shown that increasing CBF could restore evoked potential and normalize extracellular K ions.

Additional animal studies have confirmed the presence of salvageable tissue (subsequently called the penumbra) and have further refined the CBF threshold corresponding to the infarct core and to the ischemic penumbra. In 1981, Jones et al. [40] supplemented histological evidence with electrode recording sites to validate the penumbra threshold of 20 ml/100 g/min. Furthermore, they demonstrated that the core threshold, in contrast to the penumbra threshold, was time dependent.

Clinically, the use of PET in the early 1980s allowed quantitative voxel-based mapping of CMRO2 and OEF. The quantitative regional measurements were found to accurately distinguish viable from nonviable tissue. The penumbra threshold, which separates the penumbra from the oligemia, was found to be around 20 ml*100 g/min. The threshold for core, which separates the penumbra from the core, was found to be approximately 8 ml*100 g/min, which was carried out generally >3 hours from onset. However, lower thresholds characterize the core at earlier timepoints. For instance, Heiss et al. [41] showed that the volume of tissue with CBF < 12 ml/100 g/minute was still salvageable within 3 hours from onset, and the volume of salvaged penumbra correlated with neurological improvement (shown earlier by Furlan et al. [25]).

Baron et al. [42] performed PET within 18 hours of onset in a cohort of 30 patients with a first-ever middle cerebral artery stroke, and at 1 month, with co-registration of follow-up infarct from the 1-month CT scan. They replicated the Astrup and Symon model in man with identification of three distinct tissue types: the core, the ischemic penumbra, and the oligemia.

While the presence of extensive penumbra was not associated with functional outcome (reflecting the uncertain fate of the penumbra), the pattern of extensive core invariably predicts poor functional outcome, and the pattern of extensive hyperperfusion invariably predicts excellent spontaneous outcome. This key finding led the authors to advocate the use of core/penumbra imaging to triage stroke patients for individualized management and treatment.

PET studies documented that substantial volumes of penumbra persisted up to 18 hours and perhaps even beyond, suggesting that delayed treatment targeting the penumbra, including recanalization, could be considered in some patients selected based on core/penumbra imaging. The original PET studies laid the platform for the advances we see now in routine acute stroke imaging and treatment.

Despite its efficacy, PET presents with certain limitations, including cost, complexity of the procedure, relatively poor spatial resolution, limited access, the long time necessary to produce the tracers with a cyclotron and dedicated hot chemistry due to the short half-lives of the positron emitters, performing the measurements, making the use of PET in acute clinical settings impractical, and rarely clinical use.

In an attempt to transition toward more practical modalities, the interest in MRI for acute stroke was predicated on the development of diffusion-weighted imaging (DWI). The basis of DWI involves the reduction in ATPase activity that occurs almost immediately after onset of severe ischemia, which then causes a redistribution of water from the extracellular space to the intracellular space. This leads to "restricted diffusion" and reduction in the ADC, which correlates with irreversibly damaged tissue.

An early DWI study in a rat model of MCAo used the comparison of T2-weighted images and DWI for early detection of ischemia, under the principle that hyperintensity on DWI represented irreversible injury (now termed ischemic core) [43]. A few years later, it was found that the comparison of PWI and DWI was a better predictor of ischemic penumbral tissue than conventional T1 and T2 images. Within 6 hours of stroke onset, PWI had a sensitivity of 95% and a specificity of 100% in detecting the salvageable tissue. Additionally, it was reported that intermediate ADC values corresponded to penumbral tissue [44].

However, it became clear that the DWI lesion did not always reflect only ischemic core. DWI lesions have been shown to be reversible with early reperfusion, although in a fraction of cases, this reversal might be temporary with the tissue ultimately becoming infarcted [45]. Early work with PWI suggested that the ischemic penumbra was shown to correspond to the region with a mean increase of 73% in mean transit time (MTT) of the gadolinium bolus and with a 29% increase in relative cerebral blood volume (rCBV), although others suggested relative CBF was more accurate [46].

The "perfusion-diffusion mismatch" concept was coined by Warach et al. [44] and immediately gained popularity. This concept, derived from PET, postulates that salvageable tissue corresponds to the difference between the smaller diffusion lesion and the larger perfusion deficit. Consistent with previous animal and human work summarized above, mismatch incidence decreases with time, from 75% at 6 hours to 44% at 18 hours poststroke onset [47].

While these techniques have been extensively used to detect the ischemic penumbra, it was later found that the PWI/DWI mismatch region could be much larger than the true penumbra [48]. Further efforts were made to make the PWI lesion more specific for penumbra and core by directly validating PWI against PET studies of CBF [49, 50], improving perfusion algorithms, as well as applying stricter and validated perfusion thresholds. Presently, a time to maximum (Tmax) of >6 seconds is most accurate in delineating the penumbra from the core.

The shortcomings of PET and MRI were mitigated by the enhancement of the ability of CT scanners to multidetect, allowing for rapid imaging of the whole brain and the development of CT perfusions (CTP). CTP measures blood flow rather than the consequences of ischemia in tissue and attempts identification of regions of severe ischemic stress by applying thresholds for either cerebral blood volume or relative CBF. A brain tissue slab of 8–16 cm is continuously scanned over 45–90 seconds after contrast injection. Cerebral blood volume (CBV), CBF, time-to-peak (TTP), and mean transit time (MTT) are then calculated based on tissue-enhancement curves and displayed as color-coded thresholded maps, which have largely replaced qualitative eyeball techniques, to estimate CTP-based ischemic core volume.

Due to the semiquantitative CBV and CBF maps generated, CTP is very sensitive in identifying the core; however, it is not as specific for the differentiation of core and penumbra [51].

Two CTP parameters are sensitive to penumbral identification, Tmax and delay time (DT). Similar to PWI, a Tmax >6 seconds can estimate hypoperfused tissue with CBF <20 ml/100 g/min, i.e., the ischemic penumbra [52]. A DT of >2 seconds was also shown to accurately represent the penumbra and, when associated with CBF <40%, was shown to represent the core.

To aid in objective selection of patients who could benefit from thrombolysis and shorten the time process, automated measurement of MTT, Tmax, and CBF was developed, through a mathematical processing called deconvolution, with several variations [53].

MR and CT perfusion have similar accuracy in identifying key perfusion thresholds such as Tmax and DT, although CBF and CBV are less comparable. However, MRI has the clear advantage to CT in that it uses a different modality (DWI) to measure core, whereas CT relies on perfusion measures such as CBF or CBV. Nevertheless, due to the wide availability of CT scanners, CT presently is the typical assessment of acute stroke for decision-making in most centers around the world.

The importance of advanced stroke imaging is exemplified by failures of prior trials.

Earlier clinical trials utilized the aforementioned imaging modalities to visualize the core and penumbra and to extend the time windows for reperfusion treatment.

DEFUSE, an observational study involving 74 patients [54], and EPITHET, a randomized controlled trial [55], used PWI/DWI mismatch to examine the time window for tPA to 6 hours. These studies suggested that tPA improved clinical outcome and salvaged the penumbra between 3 and 6 hours of stroke onset. However, the aforementioned trials from the early 2000s suffered from lack of standardization of core and penumbral assessments.

Conducted across ten sites from August 2012 to October 2014, the Australian and New Zealand EXTEND-IA trial [56] utilized the most stringent selection criteria and was the only trial to mandate perfusion imaging, requiring evidence of salvageable tissue using the automated RAPID software (Fig. 10.3).

The criteria originally required CT perfusion mismatch for anterior circulation strokes. The hypoperfused region was defined according to a delayed arrival of an injected tracer agent (time to maximum of the residue function exceeding 6 seconds), and irreversibly injured ischemic core was estimated with the use of relative cerebral blood flow less than 30% of that in normal brain. Mismatch was defined as a ratio of greater than 1.2 between the volume of hypoperfusion and the volume of the ischemic core, an absolute difference in volume greater than 10 ml, and an ischemic core volume of less than 70 ml.

This was also the only trial to report a screening log: 7798 patients were screened, with 1044 (7%) receiving IVT and 70 (1%) receiving endovascular therapy. Out of 1044 (47%), 495

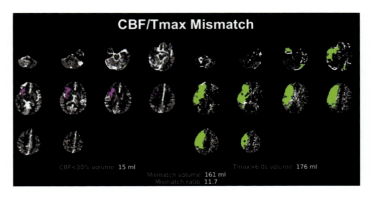

Fig. 10.3 CT perfusion scan processed by the RAPID software on a patient with a right middle cerebral artery M1 segment occlusion. On pink is the core of the infarct and on green is the tissue at risk

patients treated with IVT were excluded because their CTA did not demonstrate a large artery occlusion. It was estimated that 25% of clinically eligible patients for thrombectomy were excluded on the basis of perfusion imaging alone. All randomized patients received IVT and endovascular treatment commenced within 6 hours. This selective cohort produced excellent outcomes. The reperfusion rate was 86%, and this trial had the largest effect size, with 71% of patients in the intervention group achieving functional independence (mRS 0–2) at 90 days, compared to 40% in the control arm ($p = 0.01$, relative risk, RR 1.8). Furthermore, this trial demonstrated a large trend to mortality benefit (20 to 9%), although unlike the ESCAPE trial, the difference was not statistically significant (RR 0.4, 95% CI 0.1–1.5), probably due to the small sample size.

The criteria of CT perfusion mismatch were removed on October 12, 2016, after approximately 80 patients had been enrolled, as analysis of pooled data from other trials showed a benefit of thrombectomy in patients with larger ischemic core volumes [13]. The trial required that the ischemic-core volume be less than 70 ml only for approximately the first 80 patients, which led to the enrollment of patients with larger infarcts than in previous trials. These negative prognostic factors were expected to lead to fewer patients with an outcome of a modified Rankin scale score of 0 to 2 than were seen in the EXTEND-IA trial [3]. Among patients with acute ischemic stroke from major cerebral vessel occlusion within 4.5 hours after the onset of symptoms, intravenous tenecteplase resulted in a higher incidence of reperfusion of the occluded vascular territory before endovascular thrombectomy than did intravenous alteplase.

The SWIFT-PRIME, conducted in 39 US and European sites between December 2012 and November 2014, focused on selecting a target-mismatch penumbra profile (core <50 ml, ischemic tissue with time-to-peak of the residual function, Tmax >10 s < 100 ml, mismatch volume > 15 ml, and mismatch ratio > 1.8) using the automated RAPID penumbral imaging software. Moreover, all study centers were required to have performed at least 40 mechanical thrombectomy procedures, including at least 20 procedures with the Solitaire stent retriever, annually [57].

To identify patients with salvageable tissue, at trial launch, the selection criteria regarding imaging selection required patients to have a target-mismatch penumbral profile, with a small core of tissue that was likely to be irreversibly injured and a large region of hypoperfused tissue that was likely to be salvageable. After the first 71 eligible patients, these criteria were revised to use a small-to-moderate core-infarct strategy to accommodate study sites with limited perfusion imaging capability and to ensure accelerated treatment delivery. Patients were randomly assigned for IV t-PA to continue with t-PA alone (control group) or to undergo endovascular thrombectomy with the use of a stent retriever within 6 hours after symptom onset (intervention group). This trial had the highest rate of reperfusion (mTICI 2b/3 88%) and demonstrated improvement in functional independence (mRS 0–2) at 90 days with 60% in the intervention group versus 36% in controls (RR 1.7, 95% CI 1.23–2.33, $p < 0.001$).

The treatment and treatment response were unique in this study. The rate of substantial or complete reperfusion (88%) among patients undergoing intracranial intervention was higher in this trial than in previous trials. The high reperfusion rate is partially attributable to the more homogeneous patient population (more occlusions in the first segment of the middle cerebral artery and fewer intracranial or cervical occlusions of the internal carotid artery) and the more homogeneous intervention (an effective stent retriever and no other device classes and no intra-arterial fibrinolytic agent) in this trial than in earlier trials. The frequency of functional independence in the intervention group was high (60%) and was greater than that observed in MR CLEAN (33%) and similar to that observed in the ESCAPE trial (53%) and the EXTEND-IA trial (71%) [17]. The high frequency of this outcome probably reflects the earlier start of the intervention [23–26], the exclusion of patients with large core infarcts on the basis of imaging [27, 28], and the greater reperfusion rate in this trial.

The Highly Effective Reperfusion Evaluated in Multiple Endovascular Stroke (HERMES) trials conducted a meta-analysis of all phase 3 trials involving stent retrievers or other second-generation embolectomy devices [58, 59]. The objective was to pool the data of all the recent trials to address two questions: the degree of benefit of performing mechanical embolectomy within the established 6-hour window and whether mechanical embolectomy past 6 hours was beneficial. The HERMES authors concluded that earlier endovascular embolectomy, along with medical therapy, was associated with better functional outcome at 90 days and that this became nonbeneficial after 7.3 hours as compared to standard medical therapy alone.

Overall, the four studies were similar in methodology and presented with results that favored IAT. Additionally, they relied on referrals to experienced endovascular centers, required documentation of intracranial occlusion, and aimed at recanalization within 6 hours using stent retriever technology (82–100% overall). The main difference was that these four studies required documentation of occlusion, had a time window goal of <6 hours for recanalization, and for the most part used stent retrievers that achieved faster and more complete recanalization than previous studies. Interestingly, in a subgroup analysis, the Interventional Management of Stroke III patients with documented occlusion and similar NIHSS ranges who achieved recanalization within 6 hours also benefitted. The requirement of CTA documentation of occlusion before randomization allowed the investigators in these trials to optimize their ability to detect differences between the two groups. Moreover, the authors assured that in the patients in intervention group all had the disease they were intended to intervene on and that the control group was going to do badly without the intervention.

As the benefit of mechanical thrombectomy within 6 hours was established, the DAWN trial tested the effect of thrombectomy in patients after 6 hours from the onset of AIS. It was conducted at 26 centers in the USA, Canada, Europe, and Australia; at least 40 mechanical thrombectomy procedures had been performed at each center annually. This trial hypothesized that in patients with a clinical deficit that was disproportionately severe relative to the infarct volume, there was a chance for late thrombectomy for select patients, guided by imaging. The enrolled patients were those with occlusion of the intracranial internal carotid artery or proximal middle cerebral artery who had last been known to be well 6–24 hours earlier. Additionally, they had a mismatch between the severity of the clinical deficit and the infarct volume, which was defined according to the following criteria: those in group A were 80 years of age or older, had a score of 10 or higher on the NIHSS (scores range from 0 to 42, with higher scores indicating a more severe deficit), and had an infarct volume of less than 21 ml. The participants in group B were younger than 80 years of age, had a score of 10 or higher on the NIHSS, and had an infarct volume of less than 31 ml. Those in group C were younger than 80 years of age, had a score of 20 or higher on the NIHSS, and had an infarct volume of 31 to less than 51 ml. Infarct volume was assessed with the use of DW-MRI or CTP and was measured with the use of automated software (RAPID, iSchemaView). Patients were randomly assigned to thrombectomy plus standard care (the thrombectomy group) or to standard care alone (the control group) [60].

Enrolled patients were admitted to stroke units or intensive care units, and thrombectomy was performed with the use of the TREVO device (Stryker Neurovascular), a retrievable self-expanding stent. Rescue reperfusion therapy with other devices or pharmacologic agents was not permitted. The results demonstrated significantly improved outcomes for disability at 90 days with thrombectomy plus standard care than with standard care alone (the mean score on the utility-weighted modified Rankin scale at 90 days was 5.5 vs. 3.4 in the control group). Moreover, the trial showed that the time window for endovascular treatment may be extended to 24 hours after the patient was last known to be well, if patients are carefully selected on the basis of a disproportionately severe clinical deficit in comparison with the size of the stroke on imaging.

The Endovascular Therapy Following Imaging Evaluation for Ischemic Stroke (DEFUSE 3) trial tested the hypothesis that patients who were likely to have salvageable ischemic brain tissue, as identified by perfusion imaging, and who underwent endovascular therapy 6–16 hours after they were last known to have been well would have better functional outcomes than patients treated with standard medical therapy. In the study, a thrombectomy was performed with any FDA-approved thrombectomy device, at the discretion of the neurointerventionalist.

Patient eligibility was on the basis of if they had an initial infarct volume (ischemic core) of less than 70 ml, a ratio of volume of ischemic tissue to initial infarct volume of 1.8 or more, and an absolute volume of potentially reversible ischemia (penumbra) of 15 ml or more. Moreover, the patients were required to have an occlusion of the cervical or intracranial internal carotid artery or the proximal middle cerebral artery on CT angiography (CTA) or magnetic resonance angiography (MRA). Estimates of the volume of the ischemic core and penumbral regions from CT perfusion or MRI diffusion and perfusion scans were calculated with the use of RAPID software (iSchemaView), an automated image postprocessing system. The size of the penumbra was estimated from the volume of tissue for which there was delayed arrival of an injected tracer agent (time to maximum of the residue function [Tmax]) exceeding 6 seconds [61].

The results showed that endovascular therapy in addition to medical therapy, as compared with medical therapy alone, was associated with a favorable shift in the distribution of functional outcomes on the modified Rankin scale at 90 days (odds ratio, 2.77; $P < 0.001$) and a higher percentage of patients who were functionally independent, defined as a score on the modified Rankin scale of 0–2 (45% vs. 17%, $P < 0.001$). The 90-day mortality rate was 14% in the endovascular therapy group and 26% in the medical therapy group ($P = 0.05$), and there was no significant between-group difference in the frequency of symptomatic intracranial hemorrhage (7% and 4%, respectively; $P = 0.75$).

The development of automated core and penumbral volumetric software (including RAPID [iSchemaView, Menlo Park, CA, USA]) was a key factor contributing in the success of trials that utilized PWI/DWI and/or CTP patient selection. DEFUSE 3, DAWN, EXTEND, EXTEND-IA, and SWIFT PRIME were directly derived from the historical core/penumbra concepts, with CTP (and some MR) being the dominant selection modality in these groundbreaking trials. Together, these trials proved that perfusion imaging/core mismatch (or a clinical-core mismatch variant seen in DAWN) is efficient at selecting patients more likely to respond to reperfusion therapy.

This is especially true in the late time window trials (DAWN, DEFUSE 3, and EXTEND), where the original concept of the ischemic penumbra to select patients for therapy at late timepoints has been definitively proven. In the earlier time window studies (EXTEND-IA, SWIFT PRIME), there is still a belief that the use of perfusion imaging to select a more treatment-responsive subgroup of patients (which clearly occurred in these trials) may lead to a proportion of patients who still may benefit from being excluded.

Through these groundbreaking penumbral imaging selection studies, it can be concluded that while patients should be treated as quickly as possible, those with a favorable imaging profile (penumbra/core mismatch) have good collaterals and slow infarct growth. Such patients can achieve excellent outcomes from reperfusion therapy up to 24 hours after stroke onset.

Contemporary Strategies and Controversies in Stroke Treatment

The development of better equipment and improved devices for EVT resulted in improved rates of successful reperfusion, consistent with the post-2015 trials era. More recently, there has been a shift toward producing improved techniques and devices, improved imaging, and formulating better treatment and triage algorithms.

An important first step in this new framework was changing the medical terminology to more accurately describe AIS reperfusion. The initial nomenclature used for defining EVT success was based on cardiology imaging results; the thrombolysis in myocardial infarction score (TIMI) was converted into a cerebral circulation-based thrombolysis in cerebral infarction (TICI) score and then a "modified thrombolysis in cerebral infarction score" (mTICI), where a mTICI 2b or greater score, equivalent to >50% reperfusion of the affected territory, was considered a benchmark for successful reperfusion. This framework established a cause-and-effect relationship and allowed for the use of different methods in achieving vessel recanalization.

Multiple studies, including a meta-analysis, demonstrated the stratification of the increasingly improved reperfusion rates achieved by EVT; they elucidated that first-pass reperfusion, compared to reperfusion achieved after a first failed attempt, resulted in improved functional outcomes. These successful initial attempts have been termed first-pass effect (FPE) [62].

In the aforementioned meta-analysis, which was composed of 21 studies and 2747 patients, FPE patients had lower mortality rates than patients who did not have FPE. Moreover, further stratification endorsed that complete reperfusion with a single pass (FPE-mTICI 3) was associated with better 3-month outcomes compared with FPE-mTICI 2B (mRS 0–2, 66 vs. 46%; OR, 0.46; 95% CI, 0.037–0.57), better mortality rates (8% vs. 14%), and less intracranial hemorrhage (22% vs. 31%). This connection established between recanalization rates, FPE and clinical outcome, established a new threshold, FPE-mTICI 2B or even FPE-mTICI 2c-3, which is gaining wide acceptance as a new benchmark for evaluating thrombectomy devices. This can be attributed to the latest trials, in which devices achieve >90% reperfusion rates, and there is very little differentiating them [16–18].

Stent retrievers played a big role in the success of the six recent landmark trials, being used in more than 80% of patients [23, 24, 38–41]. Since 2015, the technology underlying stent retrievers has substantially improved. However, randomized controlled trials demonstrating a correlation between these new technologies and an improvement in recanalization, functional outcomes, and reduced complications when compared with existing stent retrievers have yet to be performed. Moreover, performance comparison has been limited mainly to historical cohorts and results achieved by landmark past studies.

Besides the Solitaire and TREVO devices mentioned above, a third-generation stent retriever is the EmboTrap reperfusion device (Neuravi/Cerenovus), which has a dual-layer structure furnished with articulating petals and a distal capture zone, which allows for a firmer grip with stronger radial force on the clot and entrapment of clot fragments generated by the EVT procedure. This device's efficacy was validated by an open-label, single-arm, multicenter, prospective clinical trial conducted by manufacturer of the device, titled "Analysis of Revascularization in Ischemic Stroke with EmboTrap (ARISE II)." This study enrolled 227 patients. The mTICI 2b reperfusion rate within three passes was 80.2%, while the final mTICI 2b reperfusion rate was 92.5%. A good functional outcome of mRS 0–2 at 90 days was achieved by 67% of the cohort, with a mortality rate of 9%, paving the way for FDA approval [63].

Another third-generation stent retriever is the three-dimensional (3D) revascularization device (Penumbra Alameda, CA, USA). A multicenter, randomized controlled trial with 198 enrolled patients was conducted to evaluate the safety and efficacy of this device in combination with an intermediate catheter. Of the 198 recruited patients, 98 underwent thrombectomy with the 3D stent retriever in conjunction with an intermediate catheter and achieved mTICI 2b-3 reperfusion in 81.9% of the patients, significantly higher than the comparison arm, where direct aspiration alone with an intermediate catheter achieved only mTICI 2b-3 reperfusion rate of 69.8% in 100 patients [64].

The Tiger retriever (Rapid Medical, Yokneam, Israel), a newer handle-controlled mechanism-based stent retriever, permits the operator to incrementally adjust the diameter of a nitinol-braided stent as well as collapse it. This feature aids in better wall apposition, robust clot integration, and a more finely controlled exertion of radial force in different vascular segments. This device is CE approved and has been studied in "The Treatment With Intent to Generate Endovascular Reperfusion" (TIGER) trial, a single-arm, prospective, multicenter study comparing the Tiger retriever to outcomes in six recent pivotal studies (TREVO 2, SWIFT, MR CLEAN, ESCAPE, REVASCAT, and SWIFT PRIME) and evaluating the Solitaire and TREVO stent retriever devices [64].

Alongside the evolution in stent retriever-based therapy was aspiration thrombectomy (AT). Also known as the contact aspiration technique, which was originally used with the Penumbra aspiration pump system (PS) in combination with a separator to break up the clot, this technique underwent gradual improvement with the introduction of stronger aspiration that was applied through larger-caliber catheters, more distally. The basis of the technique was to size the catheter to the artery without causing wedging in order to efficiently aspirate the thrombus.

Initially, a proprietary aspiration pump was used to generate a continuous negative suction of up to 20 mm Hg with the separator moved back and forth to clear the ingested clot. Later on, the forced aspiration thrombectomy (FAST) technique was used as a secondary procedure when revascularization failed with the PS separator. Manual aspiration with a 20/50 cc syringe was done through the reperfusion catheter without the separator, resulting in an improved rate of recanalization in comparison to the original PS technique.

The ADAPT ("A direct aspiration first-pass technique"), which was introduced later on, relied exclusively on the aspiration force of a pump to remove the clot. This was possible due to a newer-generation, more flexible, atraumatic large-bore, coil-reinforced catheters [65]. The larger lumens allowed for a larger surface area of contact with the clot and increased aspiration capacity. There existed two modes of clot retrieval possible: the "disrupted clot type," in which, if the clot was disrupted, blood flowed into the pump canister, and the "whole clot type," in which the lack of flow into the canister signified that the intact clot was wedged at the tip. Since crossing the occlusion is no longer necessary, the rates of neuro-thromboemboli and hemorrhage associated with superselective angiography with a microcatheter and a wire are reduced, in addition to recanalization times (as quickly as just 4.5 minutes from puncture). This technique gained popularity due to early recanalization (<35 minutes), which resulted in more complete revascularization and better clinical outcomes. Furthermore, since it allowed for an easy alternative to stent retriever techniques (usually after three failed attempts) and showed comparable rates of successful reperfusion (78% in the ADAPT-FAST trial, improving to 95% with stentriever bailout), aspiration thrombectomy challenged the monopoly of stent retriever techniques [65].

At the core of the technological advancements in catheter aspiration devices was the improved force of aspiration, directly proportional to the inner diameter (ID) of the catheter, coupled with improved navigability, thereby allowing these forces to be applied further in the cerebral vasculature tree in a safe manner. Prior scientific examination has similarly established the powerful relationship of ID to pressure loss and flow rate in small vessels. To take advantage of this principle, three new larger bore 0.071- to 0.072-in aspiration catheters were recently introduced for stroke thrombectomy. These catheters are named the Jet 7, the Vecta 71, and the React 71 and are some of the largest bore direct aspiration catheters on the market that can fit within the present guide catheters and are able to generate a larger aspiration force.

An early study looking at the navigability and efficacy of these aspiration catheters showed that they were able to reach the face of the clot in a high proportion (87%) of cases: 100% with React 71, 93% with Vecta 71, and 43% with Jet 7 ($p = 0.002$). The rate of mTICI 2b-3 reperfusion was also high in all three catheters and was achieved in 92% of cases: 95% with React 71, 89% with Jet 7, and 89% with Vecta 71. These large-bore catheters achieved a 39% FPE rate in this small series. The efficacy of aspiration catheters, combined with shorter procedural times and cost-effectiveness, led to the development of even larger bore aspiration catheters. In fact, several 8 F 0.088-in (I.D.) aspiration catheters have been shown to be feasible in navigating preclinical models of the middle cerebral artery M1 segment and the basilar artery and to be superior in clot extraction compared with smaller bore catheters.

In an effort to address other elements of the physical forces generating thromboaspiration for stroke thrombectomy, the pump activation mode was developed. In a change from the typical static continuous vacuum, either with a pump or a large syringe, the concept of cyclical aspiration was introduced. Using a SOFIA Plus catheter (MicroVention Inc., Aliso Viejo, CA), either a static (29 inHg) or cyclical (18–29 inHg, 0.5 Hz) aspiration was employed using the digital CLEAR Aspiration System (Insera Therapeutics, Sacramento, CA), and eight thrombus aspiration experiments were conducted for each aspiration type in a flow model.

The study highlighted that by varying the pressure dynamics through cyclical aspiration, there was an increased aspiration force on the occlusion, resulting in more successful clot clearance when compared with static aspiration. This may be attributed to the initial clot softening from dynamic compression or to dynamic friction being less than the static friction that occurs when the thrombus is stuck at the tip of the catheter. This concept was tested and confirmed in a different study using various types of catheters with different inner diameters (0.054–0.088 in). In this study, the use of cyclic aspiration (18–29 inHg, 0.5 Hz) resulted in better clot ingestion into the aspiration catheter and effectively reduced the rate of distal emboli.

These two MT recanalization methods were compared against each other in the Contact Aspiration vs. Stent Retriever for Successful Revascularization (ASTER) study. This was a randomized, open-label, blinded end point superiority clinical trial designed to address this problem. In this trial, 381 patients were enrolled, with 192 patients assigned to first-line direct aspiration and 189 assigned to first-line stent retriever use. Successful reperfusion was achieved at similar rates with direct aspiration (85.4%) and stent retrievers (83.1%), $p = 0.53$. Nonetheless, trial was underpowered and failed to demonstrate a significant difference between the two techniques.

After the failure of the ASTER trial, the similar reperfusion rates between modalities led a North American group to change track and conduct a noninferiority trial in 15 North American sites. The goal was to once again compare the efficacy between large-bore direct aspiration and stent retrievers. Titled COMPASS, this trial featured 270 patients without a large early infarct core (ASPECTS>6) and who presented within 6 hours of onset. Ultimately, 134 received direct aspiration as first-line treatment and 136 received stent retriever use as first-line treatment. Direct aspiration achieved 52% good functional outcomes at 3 months, which was comparable with the 50% achieved by first-line stent retriever use and reached noninferiority in the analysis ($p = 0.0014$). This trial was the landmark trial to provide level 1 evidence in support of direct aspiration. Moreover, the authors stated that even in the event of failure of direct aspiration, the large-bore catheter was still at the clot face and that a stent retriever could be quickly deployed over the thrombus. This led to a significantly shorter procedural duration in the initial direct aspiration arm when compared with stent retriever use. An additional benefit noted was the cost-effectiveness of aspiration catheters.

Considering this new evidence, the 2019 AHA/ASA updated the guidelines for stroke management assigned to ADAPT a level of I B-R (moderate quality of evidence) [4]. In addition, the SNIS Standards and Guidelines Committee [5] confirmed MT guidelines for posterior circulation stroke.

Acknowledging the huge heterogeneity in both clot and patient characteristics and the fact that there is no single "silver bullet" which would prove superior in all cases, Kang et al., in 2013, codified the concept of a switching strategy to maximize the technical outcome. This was defined as the change from one EVT technique to another after angiographic recanalization failure, later renamed as the *switching/bailout technique.*

In switching from stent retriever thrombectomy to aspiration, two possible options are available. The first option involves removal of the microcatheter-stent retriever combination completely and then introducing the aspiration catheter as usual similar to primary ADAPT. The second option is to only remove the stent retriever while leaving the microcatheter in place. The following step is to pass the microwire with a docking wire and use this to exchange the aspiration system directly into place. This latter option provides utility if navigation is difficult.

The second option features switching from aspiration to stent retriever thrombectomy, so that an additional microcatheter wire can be navigated through the indwelling aspiration catheter for subsequent delivery of the stent retriever.

Unlike in the bailout technique, where methods were switched in the case of failure, smaller observational studies showed very high reperfusion rates and excellent functional outcome for combined approaches, as methods of MT were combined to work concomitantly.

This was facilitated by an extension of the mode through which thrombectomy is presently applied. Stent retrievers are introduced through a *guide catheter system (GC)*, which usually features a large bore (8–9 F), and are divided into three types: conventional guide catheters (CGC), distal access catheters (DAC), and balloon guide catheters (BGCs).

An exchange method or coaxial advancement technique is used to place the GC. The tip is usually parked at the ICA bulb or V1/V2 segments [50]. Generally, CGCs such as Neuron or Envoy are better suited in the posterior circulation, while DACs require a triaxial system and are of use in more distal occlusions or tortuous vessels. Both DAC and CGC are brought as close to the occlusion as possible to reduce the retrieval corridor and thrombus dispersion. The efficiency of aspiration, however, is reduced due to their narrower lumens.

The advantage of BGCs, a simple upgrade from the typical guide catheter with a large lumen, is an inflatable balloon on the distal tip of the catheter, over the other two other GCs, which creates both flow arrest and flow reversal distal to the balloon. This permits more efficient aspiration and reduced rates of neuro-thromboemboli (10–12% vs. 53% with BGC).

The benefits of BGC thrombectomy have been indicated in multiple different studies. The investigator-initiated TRACK registry, which audits the TREVO device, featured 536 anterior circulation stroke patients, of whom 279 (52.1%) had BGC placement, and showed that mTICI 2b-3 scores were higher in the BGC group (84% vs. 75.5%; $p = 0.01$) with improved 3-month outcomes (57% vs. 40%; $p = 0.0004$) and mortality rates (13% vs. 23%; $p = 0.008$). This was despite the fact that aspiration catheter or intermediate catheter use was more common in the non-BGC group [35]. In the NASA and STRATIS registries (Systematic Evaluation of Patients Treated with Neurothrombectomy Devices for Acute Ischemic Stroke), a similar effect was seen for 3-month functional outcomes. More specifically, in these two registries, the FPE was more often seen with the use of a BGC. A meta-analysis of studies with BGC use, which included 2022 patients, demonstrated that BGC use was in fact associated with a higher chance of FPE (OR, 2.1; 95% CI, 1.65–2.55).

As BCGs and large-bore distal aspiration catheters presented specific compatibility challenges, the industry was focused on designing novel aspiration catheters that would be compatible with their BCGs (e.g., novel 7 F Catalyst fits into 8 F Flowgate or

Flowgate2 BGC). The ASTER trial documented a trend toward better mTICI 3 and better clinical outcomes in BGC-treated patients, using direct aspiration.

Aside from aspiration, stent retrievers, and a combination of the two, additional methods include distal-protection devices and rescue stenting. The "Lazarus effect cover-assisted MT" is a distal embolization protection device for stent retriever thrombectomy. It features a funnel-shaped nitinol mesh designed to surround the stent retriever and the enmeshed thrombus during retrieval.

Following stent retriever deployment, the Lazarus device is positioned at its proximal end, and the retraction of the stent retriever against the device results in it inverting and rolling over the outside of the stent retriever. This protective sheath presumably prevents clot fragmentation and distal embolization and has also been used with distal aspiration techniques.

Another method is "rescue stenting." While it is uncommonly used due to reperfusion rates in AIS LVO being in the 90% range, it is practical for a subset of patients in whom recanalization fails. One of the key reasons for failure of EVT is underlying intracranial atherosclerotic stenosis (ICAS). ICAS is routinely diagnosed during the EVT procedure by repeated recanalization and then acute reocclusion of the vessel. In a Korean series of failed EVTs, this occurred in up to 77% of the patients. Presently, no guidelines exist for the optimum treatment in patients who failed thrombectomy. An alternate technique is to perform permanent stenting in an attempt to preserve the patency of the vessel.

The effectiveness of "rescue stenting" was demonstrated in an initial study of 45 failed thrombectomy patients, where the 17 patients with rescue stenting had better outcomes and less cerebral herniation than the 28 non-stenting patient [61]. This technique was validated in a large retrospective analysis of patients from 16 Korean stroke centers. In this study, patients with anterior circulation LVOs who failed to recanalize following EVT were split into rescue stenting and non-rescue stenting groups. Out of the 148 failed EVT patients, 48 received rescue stenting and 100 did not. Subsequent results show that 31 out of 48 rescue stenting patients (64.6%) had successful mTICI 2b-3 reperfusion with rescue stenting, while none of the 100 patients without rescue stenting achieved reperfusion. Good functional outcome at 3 months was observed in 39.6% of the rescue stenting group and in 22.0% of the non-rescue stenting group ($p = 0.031$) without an increase in SICH or mortality. Moreover, in the rescue stenting group with successful reperfusion, 54.8% achieved good outcome despite the initial EVT failure, equivalent to the functional outcomes with mTICI 2b-3 reperfusion in the initial EVT attempts of 55.4%.

A meta-analysis on rescue stenting, which included articles from 2015 to 2019, supported these results. In a sample of 352 patients, there was improved outcomes in the stenting arm compared with the refractory occlusion arm (OR, 2.87; 95% CI, 1.77–4.66; $p < 0.001$; I2, 0%) with reduced mortality, but there was some heterogeneity between studies for mortality (OR, 0.39; 95% CI, 0.16–0.93; $p = 0.03$; I2, 43%).

In a recent multinational study on emergency rescue stenting in AIS involving seven neurovascular centers, good outcome was observed in 73 out of 163 (44.8%) patients with recorded outcomes at 90 days. This is considerably better than the rates of 7–22% found in cohorts with reocclusion or persistent occlusion reports without rescue stenting. However, the rate of SICH in this analysis (11%) was higher than in the aggregated thrombectomy studies without intracranial stenting of 4.4%, and this was more common in anterior circulation occlusions than posterior circulation occlusions. A lower number of thrombectomy attempts before rescue stenting were correlated with better functional outcomes.

The decision to perform rescue stenting is complex, as the permanent placement of a stent requires either acute glycoprotein 2b/3a inhibitors or dual antiplatelet treatment to prevent acute reocclusion due to in-stent thrombosis. In acute stroke patients with already sizable amounts of ischemic or infarcted tissue, these medications contribute to a potentially higher risk of symptomatic intracranial hemorrhage. Presently, there is limited data and a lack of consensus regarding antiplatelet management for intracranial stenting during thrombectomy.

As can be concluded from the heterogeneous nature of LVO AIS, there are still concerns unanswered by the guidelines. These imminent questions describe subsets of patients who are still frequently encountered and for whom future studies would elucidate the best treatment algorithm.

Large Ischemic Core

While the present guidelines clearly indicate that EVT should be performed for patients without a large early infarct or with an ASPECTS of six or more, there exists a substantial proportion of patients who present to the hospital with an AIS with a sizable ischemic core. While the evidence is unclear, these patients may still derive some benefit from EVT. Pending the outcomes of randomized controlled trials, core-lab adjudicated pooled analyses of existing studies may shed preliminary insight into this crucial question.

In a study pooling data from seven randomized trials with a total of 1764 patients, of which 871 were in the EVT arm and 893 in the best medical treatment arm, it was indicated that EVT was associated with better functional outcomes across a wide range of pretreatment imaging types on ordinal shift analyses [64]. This included all ASPECTS groups, except for ASPECTS 0–2, in which the low sample size was not statistically significant. However, this should be interpreted with caution, as in patients with a large ischemic burden or ASPECTS 4 or less, EVT was associated with significantly more SICH.

Similarly, a secondary analysis of the Optimizing Patient Selection for Endovascular Treatment in Acute Ischemic Stroke (SELECT) trial demonstrated that EVT was associated with better functional independence (mRS 0–2) compared with medical management alone (OR, 3.27; 95% CI, 1.11–9.62; $p = 0.03$). Moreover, EVT was also associated with less infarct growth and smaller final infarct volume than medical treatment [66]. These aforementioned analyses provide a strong evidence to support further investigation of the use of EVT for patients with large infarcts and poor ASPECTS at baseline.

The preliminary results from these studies led to the ongoing SELECT-2 trial, which was designed to evaluate thrombectomy compared with medical management in distal ICA and MCA M1 occlusions with a large core on either CT (ASPECTS 3–5) or advanced perfusion imaging (rCBF <30% or ADC < 620 or 50 ml or more). The tentative completion date of this trial is at the end of 2021 [67]. Other ongoing clinical trials, such as TENSION (NCT03094715), TESLA (NCT03805308), and IN EXTREMIS [68, 69], are also actively recruiting patients and will provide conclusive evidence on the use of EVT in patients with a large ischemic core at presentation [67].

Clinically Mild Strokes with LVO

Another subset of patients are those who present with LVOs but mild strokes clinically. These scenarios are typically defined at NIHSS threshold of <5, where the risk of the EVT procedure needs to be weighed carefully against the potential benefit. A pooled data analysis was conducted featuring six comprehensive stroke centers with 300 patients having LVO and NIHSS 0–5, with 80 patients undergoing EVT and 220 patients undergoing best medical therapy [70]. The best medical treatment group allowed for rescue EVT if there was subsequent neurological deterioration. While the groups were not similar, EVT was associated with better functional outcomes (OR, 3.1; 95% CI, 1.4–6.9), and in a propensity-matched analysis, the superiority of EVT over best medical treatment persisted (84.4% vs. 70.1%; $P = 0.03$) [64].

Recently, another meta-analysis pooled patient data from 16 centers from 2013 to 2017. This study evaluated 251 patients with LVO and mild stroke, of which 138 were treated with EVT and 113 with best medical treatment. The results demonstrated that the 3-month functional outcomes were better in the best medical treatment group when compared with the EVT group (77.4% vs. 88.5%; $p = 0.02$) [37]. The rate of asymptomatic ICH was also lower in the best medical management group as compared with the EVT group (4.6% vs. 17.5%; $p = 0.002$). Moreover, there was no difference in the rate of reperfusion or in safety outcomes between the two groups [64, 66, 71].

It is expected that future RCTs will further elucidate if mild strokes with LVO should be treated via EVT. One of these RCTs is ENDOLOW, which is studying anterior circulation occlusions with NIHSS scores 0–5 and is enrolling patients in Canada, the USA, Germany, and Sweden. The INEXTREMIS trial also features a sub-study that is evaluating ischemic stroke patients with an NIHSS<6 and LVO occlusions and aims to answer this important question [71].

Very Late Presenting Patients: Acute Stroke Beyond 24 Hours

Recent evidence from the AURORA study, which pooled data from six randomized trials to examine effect of EVT in anterior circulation proximal LVO stroke from 6 to 24 h from time last seen well, suggests a potential benefit of EVT in achieving reduced disability on functional outcome in terms of mRS in this group of patients, with an adjusted common odds ratio of 2.54 (95% CI, 1.82–3.54; $p < 0.0001$). Moreover, the number needed to treat to reduce mRS by 1 point was three patients. Furthermore, no significant differences in mortality or SICH were seen between EVT and control groups [72]. This further validates the results of previous trials, which supported the fact that carefully selected patients benefit from thrombectomy up to 24 hours [61, 73].

However, there is another subset of patients who present after 24 hours. Presently, no clinical trials or guidelines detailing how we can manage these patients exist. Kim et al. studied the benefit of EVT in patients presenting very late [74]. In a subgroup analysis of 150 patients, who presented more than 16 h from their last known well time, EVT was performed only in 24 patients, but a propensity-matched analysis showed it was associated with increased odds of having favorable functional recovery at 3 months (adjusted OR, 11.08; 95% CI, 1.88–108.60). In a further subgroup of patients 24 hours from last known well, EVT was associated with favorable outcomes as well (adjusted OR, 10.54; 95% CI, 2.18–59.34) [75]. These preliminary studies provide evidence in support of a possibility of maintaining the penumbra beyond 24 hours in patients with good collaterals [74].

Direct to Thrombectomy Table: No IV tPA

Timing directly impacts the functional outcome in acute stroke thrombectomy, as any delay in treatment initiation negatively impacts patients' functional outcomes [67, 76]. While IV-tPA can recanalize acute stroke occlusions, EVT has shown higher rate of recanalization. Hence, there is now a school of thought that instead of administering IV tPA, whether at an intervening primary stroke center or the comprehensive stroke center, patients with AIS from an LVO should be treated with EVT.

The SKIP trial, a RCT carried out in Japan, enrolled 200 AIS patients with anterior circulation occlusions presenting within 4 hours of onset [68]. At 3 months, the rate of good functional outcome was similar between the direct thrombectomy (59%) and combined bridging approach (57%). Moreover, both groups were found to have a similar mortality rate. However, this trial was unable to prove noninferiority of direct to thrombectomy over bridging IV tPA (0.6 mg/kg Japanese standardized dose), attributable to it being underpowered with a modest sample size. While the rate of asymptomatic hemorrhage and SICH did not significantly differ between both arms, the combined rate of any ICH was significantly lower for the EVT group.

Two other trials, similar in design to the SKIP trial were conducted in China, across multiple stroke centers, also studied bridging IV tPA in thrombectomy. The DIRECT-MT trial, with 656 enrolled patients, revealed that endovascular thrombectomy alone was noninferior to combined intravenous alteplase and endovascular thrombectomy when considering the functional outcome at 90 days (adjusted common odds ratio, 1.07; 95% confidence interval, 0.81–1.40; $p = 0.04$ for noninferiority). In addition, the noninferiority margin was set at a high value of 20% margin of confidence in this trial. The noninferiority test in the DEVT trial also highlighted that the endovascular thrombectomy alone was noninferior to the combined IV thrombolysis and endovascular thrombectomy group ($z = 2.7157$, p for noninferiority = 0.003) [69, 70]. This trial was terminated after the first interim analysis in May 2020 due to the outcome measured having surpassed the prespecified efficacy boundary. In this study, there was no significantly different rate of symptomatic ICH between groups; however, the rate of any ICH is significantly higher in the bridging r-TPA and thrombectomy group. It is worth noting that given these trials were performed in East Asian populations, further evidence is needed in a more diverse population. The SWIFT-DIRECT, MR CLEAN NOIV, and DIRECT-SAFE trials are upcoming international RCTs that can fulfill this role as they aim to provide more information on the adoption of thrombectomy alone approach against bridging IV tPA [70].

Tandem Occlusions

A tandem occlusion (TO) is a thromboembolic obstruction in the intracranial cerebral vasculature in combination with an extracranial carotid artery occlusion. It can occur in up to one-sixth of ischemic stroke patients [37]. Typically, TOs do not have good recanalization rates with IV tPA, and therefore EVT is suggested [22]. In fact, subgroup analyses of the ESCAPE and MR CLEAN studies indicated that patients with TO have better outcomes with early or concurrent treatment of the extracranial occlusion rather than later in a staged procedure [77, 78]. Nonetheless, there is a lack of consensus on the optimal endovascular procedure for acute TO.

The present issue pertains to the best method of treating TO in acute stroke. The point of contention is if it is better to initially bypass the extracranial occlusion and remove the intracranial occlusion first before returning to tackle the extracranial stenosis (the "retrograde" approach) or if it is preferable to attempt primary recanalization of the extracranial occlusion first before moving on to treat the intracranial occlusion (the "antegrade" approach). The antegrade approach uses primary stenting to jail the extracranial stenotic atheromatous plaque, thereby preventing distal emboli [78]. One potential drawback of the antegrade approach is the procedural time used for carotid stent placement, as it creates a delay in the time to intracranial reperfusion, possibly resulting in an increase of the final infarct volume [75, 79]. Furthermore, stent retriever-based thrombectomy techniques have the potential of entanglement between the struts of the stent retriever and carotid stent during withdrawal if the guiding catheter cannot be advanced through the carotid stent. Moreover, the retrograde approach achieves intracranial recanalization faster, and some purport that this gives better functional outcomes [75]; however, it may be difficult to pass through the proximal occlusion, and subsequent emboli from the proximal occlusion can sometimes reocclude the intracranial circulation.

Type of Anesthesia for Thrombectomy

For patients treated with EVT particularly, anesthesia has indicated benefits, especially when considering complex anatomy, difficult cases, or restless and aphasic patients. The type of anesthesia used may impact the success outcomes for mechanical thrombectomy. General anesthesia (GA) may improve procedural safety preventing body movement as well as protecting the airway, while conscious sedation (CS) allows for neurologic monitoring with hemodynamic stability and a quicker puncture time [80]. Due to the lack of a consensus in the present literature, a preference for which type of anesthesia to use is undetermined.

Initial retrospective studies often based their anesthesia choice on patient characteristics and the comfort level of the administrator. A retrospective study featuring 1174 patients from 2009 to 2013 concluded that GA was inferior to CS; however, there was limited data on the important factors such as blood pressure and the NIHSS. Furthermore, their outcomes studied were only mortality and length of stay [80]. Conversely, another retrospective database study of 2512 patients concluded the opposite: that CS was superior to GA for stroke interventions [81].

Intra-arterial Neuroprotection, Middle Vessel Occlusion, and AI-Powered Tools in AIS: New Frontiers

A deeper understanding of the use of EVT for AIS treatment presents an opportunity to address multiple prevention and treatment aspects, attributable to the various technological innovations combined with extensive data on patients and interventions, and unprecedented computing processing. In this chapter, we focus specifically on potential innovative directions in endovascular invasive therapies which could drive future AIS treatment.

Stroke Secondary to Distal Medium-Vessel Occlusion

Distal medium-vessel occlusion (DMVO) recanalization presents further challenges to vessel recanalization, despite significantly improved LVO recanalization rates. Around 35–40% of AIS cases occur due to LVO, while 25–40% are caused by medium-vessel occlusions (MeVOs). Characterized by distal occlusion location and less ischemia, MeVO strokes have better outcomes when compared with LVO strokes, but cohort studies indicate that the outcomes are frequently poor, despite best medical management [82].

The exact definition of a medium-sized vessel also requires consensus, as vessel size and anatomy may be subjected to interobserver variability. MeVO was defined as an occlusion of the M2/M3 middle cerebral artery/A2/A3 anterior cerebral artery and P2/P3 posterior cerebral artery segments in a study with pooled data from two multicenter prospective cohorts. In this study, only 50.0% of patients with DMVO achieved an excellent outcome (mRS score, 0–1) at 90 days, and 67.4% achieved an independent outcome (mRS score, 0–2). Moreover, the authors found that intravenous alteplase was significantly associated with lower mRS scores in mRS shift analysis, but no significant association with excellent outcome (mRS score, 0–1) was noted.

Moreover, even in the alteplase group, early recanalization was achieved in <50% of study cohort, suggesting insufficient efficacy of intravenous alteplase as a stand-alone treatment for DMVO strokes [83].

Data from a preliminary meta-analysis of 12 nonrandomized studies indicated that EVT for patients with occlusions of M2 segment of middle cerebral artery that can be safely accessed is associated with high recanalization rates and good clinical outcomes [84].

Until recently, endovascular treatment of DMVO was considered to have a high risk-benefit ratio with less severe clinical deficits and increased risk of iatrogenic complications. Additionally, the isolated nature of deficits associated with these and other MeVOs (A2/A3/M3/P2/P3) such as abulia, quadrantanopia, aphasia, and ataxia makes NIHSS-based and protocolized patient selection challenging (Fig. 10.4).

Determining the infarct core and penumbra accurately in MeVO stroke may be challenging or not possible at all, as recent literature suggests that we presently lack the ability to precisely delineate infarct "core" with the commonly used imaging modali-

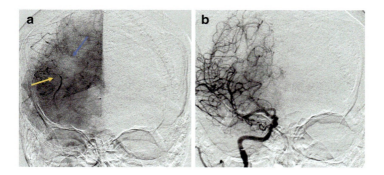

Fig. 10.4 Patient who presented with a distal right middle cerebral artery occlusion. (**a**) Initial injection of the right internal carotid artery, parenchymal phase, demonstrates an occlusion of a distal right middle cerebral artery branch (M3/4) (yellow arrow) resulting in an area of lack of parenchymal blood flow (blue arrow). (**b**) Patient underwent aspiration thrombectomy resulting in recanalization of the occluded branch

ties [85]. More importantly, delineating ischemic core and penumbra may be of importance, as previous early time window LVO trials failed to demonstrate any volume cutoff below which EVT was no longer beneficial. Moreover, present EVT guidelines for LVO patients in the early time window exclusively rely on NCCT ASPECTS to estimate the degree of irreversible tissue damage [86]. Despite this, using ASPECTS in MeVO stroke may be problematic, since the anterior and posterior cerebral artery territories are not represented at all.

Given the deficit severity and improvement in the tools to overcome these technical challenges, such as smaller and more flexible aspiration catheters coupled with more finely controlled mini stentrievers, the potential benefit of EVT in patients with dominant M2 occlusions is still considerable. However, there are numerous technical challenges that are presented with EVT for MeVO stroke. At the present stage, the risk of vasospasm and dissection when the catheter size matches or exceeds the vessel diameter, which can happen with large-bore aspiration catheters in MeVOs, is unknown. Moreover, medium-sized vessels can be too small to harbor a regular-sized distal access catheter (DAC), as most of the presently used DACs are 5–6 F in diameter.

Furthermore, the DAC often gets stuck at the ledge of a bifurcation point, such as the M1 bifurcation; however, this ledge effect can be overcome through the use of wedge-shaped microcatheters. Lastly, using a primary combined approach (i.e., the combination of stent retriever, DAC, and balloon guide catheter) and advancing the system in a triaxial manner, as it is commonly done for LVOs, may not be possible because of insufficient catheter length and diameter discrepancies. For example, using a longer DAC to access an M3 occlusion may not allow for a small enough and long enough microcatheter capable of deploying a stent. Thus, presently, the microwire and microcatheter are often introduced without a DAC. Once the microcatheter is in place, the stent can be deployed, and the microcatheter removed before the distal access catheter is navigated to the site of occlusion (socalled blind exchange mini-pinning technique) [87, 88].

Perez-Garcia et al. [89] addressed this issue by comparing the safety and efficacy of EVT using mini stent retrievers alone (used earlier in the study period) versus mini stent retrievers combined with low-profile distal aspiration catheters through the blind exchange/mini-pinning (BEMP) technique in patients with MeVO in M2/M3/A1/A2/A3/P1 and distal posterior cerebral artery segments. The authors studied the procedural, safety (emboli to unwanted territories and hemorrhagic complications), and clinical outcomes. Out of the 102 enrolled patients (106 MeVO in different arteries), 56 were treated with the BEMP technique, and 50 were treated with the mini stent retriever alone. The authors found improved outcomes with the BEMP technique, including a higher rate of first-pass extended thrombolysis in cerebral ischemia 2c/3 recanalization (57% vs. 34%) and lower rates of rescue therapy (7.1% vs. 22%). Multivariable logistic regression analysis demonstrated the BEMP technique to be the sole independent factor associated with first-pass recanalization, with no difference in mortality or functional independence between the groups. Moreover, although clinical outcomes were comparable in both groups, mini stent retriever technique was associated with an unacceptably high rate of emboli to new territory (1.8% vs. 12%) and symptomatic intracerebral hemorrhage (1.9% vs. 12.8%). For future studies replicating this, patient selection is crucial, especially identifying patients with an M2 occlusion.

The need for a specialized technique to allow distal catheter repositioning is a temporary problem, as many of the newer stent retrievers can be deployed through a 017 microcatheter and more microcatheters are now available in 160 cm length. In contrast, numerous authors reported promising results of primary aspiration as the first-line approach in MeVO stroke, which may constitute an equally effective alternative to stent retriever-based techniques [87, 90–94]. However, a thorough and unbiased comparison of different MeVO EVT techniques in future trials is vital for validating either of these approaches.

The use of specialized devices, specifically developed for thrombectomy of MeVOs, is important. However, these devices present with the challenges of accounting for operator experience, especially when considering the constant development of even newer devices. Moreover, the selection of functional and safety outcomes for the MeVO population needs to be specific. While a good functional outcome is acceptable for LVO population, defining primary outcome as 90-day mRS score of 0–2 is impractical and suboptimal for patients with MeVO. Domain-specific outcome measures or quality of life assessments can also be considered for these trials. Furthermore, since the median presenting NIHSS score is much lower in these patients, the traditionally used ECASS (European Cooperative Acute Stroke Study) and SITS-MOST (Safe Implementation of Thrombolysis in Stroke-Monitoring Study) definitions of symptomatic intracerebral hemorrhage outcome for patients with LVO need modification to account for lesser clinical worsening in NIHSS that might be seen in patients with MeVO.

Similarly, the definitions of early neurological recovery need appropriate modifications. It is hoped that these randomized trials will parallel those that established EVT as standard of care for anterior circulation LVO, thereby shifting the treatment paradigm for patients with MeVO that would subsequently improve patient outcomes. Lastly, it is important to recognize that direct aspiration thrombectomy in distal vessels, such as the M3 or M4, carries a risk of avulsion injury to the perforators, and therefore further studies are needed to determine their safety and effectiveness. Presently, there is a belief that that reperfusion rates with EVT could improve further with the use of smaller diameter next-generation stent retrievers and aspiration devices.

Intra-arterial Neuroprotection

Neuroprotection to prevent infarct progression as a potential treatment for AIS is associated with a rather lackluster history. The failures of these prior neuroprotection trials may be attributable to problems with the preclinical assessment of these drugs and the design/implementation of clinical trials.

Several approaches, including nonpharmacological ones, to freeze the penumbra and minimize expansion of core volume are presently being tested in the laboratory and clinical trials. The endovascular technique in stroke enables, without any additional manipulation, the potential for infusion of drugs directly into the region at risk. Aside from convenience, there are multiple potential advantages to delivering neuroprotective therapy via the intra-arterial route. Hence, in stroke cases, providing neuroprotective therapy via the IA route could provide a high concentration of drug directly to the target ischemic territory while simultaneously avoiding first-pass metabolism and limiting systemic toxicity. Based on IA given in chemotherapy and vasospasm treatment, it can be noted that this has the potential to significantly improve the effectiveness of therapy compared to intravenous treatment.

Only a fraction of the neuroprotective agents tested via the intravenous, oral, or intraperitoneal route have been tested via intra-arterial delivery [95]. Specifically, there is interest in magnesium ions, which provide a physiologic noncompetitive voltage-dependent block of the NMDA receptor ion channel [96]. Moreover, additional neuroprotective benefits include promoting vasodilation and thereby increasing cerebral blood flow, inhibiting presynaptic release of excitatory neurotransmitters, blocking other voltage-gated calcium channels, antagonizing endothelin-1 and other vasoconstrictors, and replenishing an ischemia-induced Mg-deficient state [96].

The FAST-MAG trial, in which a 4 g loading dose of $MgSO_4$ was administered in the field to stroke patients, was a prominent stroke trial. Patients brought in by paramedics, followed by administering a 16 g maintenance infusion in the hospital, demonstrated feasibility with a mean serum Mg level of 3.6 mEq/L and safety with no observed drug-related major adverse events; However, there was no demonstration of efficacy. There is only one ongoing phase 1 human clinical trial in which the investigators aim to deliver IA magnesium sulfate in patients undergoing endovascular stroke intervention (NCT01502761) [28]. This study design includes four groups of five patients. The primary outcome is serum magnesium concentration, and the secondary outcome is the number of patients with serious procedure-related adverse events [95].

Similar to magnesium, verapamil, an L-type calcium channel blocker, is thought to have neuroprotective effects by reducing calcium influx into cells and thus limiting excitotoxicity. There is extensive experience in the literature of administering verapamil via IA delivery into the ICA for cerebral vasospasm, making it an attractive potential agent due to its established safety profile. Fraser et al. then followed these experiments up with a phase 1 clinical trial entitled Superselective Administration of VErapamil During Recanalization in Acute Ischemic Stroke (SAVER-I) (NCT02235558). Subjects undergoing mechanical thrombectomy with thrombolysis in cerebral infarction (TICI) 2a or better recanalization received 10 mg verapamil in 20 cc of normal saline over 20 minutes via microcatheter injection directly into the previously occluded artery. Eleven patients were included, and IA delivery was technically successful in all. The authors concluded that the IA delivery of verapamil immediately following thrombectomy is safe and feasible [95, 97].

Hypothermia has been suggested to be the most potent neuroprotective strategy given its ability to target multiple pathways simultaneously by several mechanisms within the ischemic and reperfusion cascades. Presently, it is the only neuroprotective treatment that has proven efficacy and been introduced into clinical practice to reduce hypoxic brain injury after cardiac arrest. The mechanisms by which therapeutic hypothermia provides neuroprotection are manifold, such as a reduction of cerebral brain metabolic demands and reduced infarct size. In addition, surface cooling methods are limited by increased shivering and skin necrosis. Certain previous methods have resulted in either insufficient cooling of the brain (cooling helmets and nasal cooling, limited by slow rates of temperature reduction and local cooling), while other methods (such as endovascular catheters inserted into the femoral or subclavian veins) are limited by the risks of infection, bleeding, and thrombosis as well as systemic complications. Therefore, an interest in intracarotid infusion of cold saline in order to produce a targeted, local hypothermia of the brain with less overall systemic temperature reduction is indicated [95, 98].

In 2007, a mathematical model showed that an intracarotid infusion of cold saline at a rate of 30 ml/minute can reduce brain temperature to 33–34_C in 10 minutes. The degree of the temperature drop was proportional to the rate of infusion. The feasibility, safety, and effectiveness of intracarotid infusion of cold saline for neuroprotection with targeted hypothermia have been supported and demonstrated in several animal models; this technique has been attempted in two small-scale phase 1 human clinical trials.

A 2010 US study delivered saline at 15 °C and 7 °C into the internal carotid artery (ICA) of 18 patients undergoing follow-up routine angiograms at 33 ml/minute for 10 minutes. The jugular bulb temperatures demonstrated a drop of 0.84 °C, compared to 0.15 °C for bladder temperatures. Three of the patients experienced shivering, but the vitals, neurologic exam, discomfort, and laboratory values, such as hematocrit, remained stable.

In a phase 1 study done in 2016 in China, the authors administered 4 °C saline at 30 ml/minute for 10 minutes into the ICA of 26 stroke patients undergoing thrombectomy. The rectal temperature decreased by 0.1 °C, and vitals, electrolytes, and hematocrit remained relatively unaltered during or after treatment. Therefore, the authors concluded that intra-arterial infusion of 4 °C saline following thrombectomy for LVO patients is safe and feasible [99].

The future of neuroprotection in stroke will likely involve combination therapy utilizing multiple agents. Presently, one completed phase 1 clinical trial (SAVER-I) has demonstrated the safety and feasibility of IA delivery of neuroprotective drugs immediately after reperfusion in large vessel occlusion ischemic stroke patients. Two additional clinical trials are ongoing. Furthermore, two published human clinical pilot studies have supported the safety and feasibility of infusing cold saline directly into the carotid artery in patients undergoing angiograms and in stroke patients. As additional clinical trials come to fruition, the safety profile of these techniques will become established, and the ideal ratio for neuroprotection will need to be reassessed [99, 100].

Another alternative for neuroprotection in AIS is augmentation of collateral circulation. In experimental ischemia, middle cerebral artery occlusion (MCAO) induces redistribution of cerebral blood flow (CBF) and engagement of the leptomeningeal collateral vessels. The degree of CBF redistribution is demonstrated by the size and number of pial collaterals in both experimental ischemia models and patients with LVOs. Blood flow augmentation in leptomeningeal anastomosis (LMA) can significantly influence outcomes.

Several authors have reported the strong association between robust collateral circulation and favorable outcomes following successful recanalization of LVOs. Moreover, another important piece of evidence in LMA physiology is that in acute ischemia even the most robust collateral circulation is not permanent.

Nonpharmacologic neuroprotection to slow down core expansion and preserve penumbral tissue may complement pharmacologic measures and can be minimally invasive and easy to administer.

Among endovascular approaches, transient descending aortic balloon occlusion to increase perfusion in the brain that has been tested in rodents with positive results was attempted in the past. The SENTIS phase 2b trial (Safety and Efficacy of NeuroFlo Technology in Ischemic Stroke) demonstrated the safeness of this approach but not its efficacy [101]. However, once again, candidates for reperfusion therapies were excluded. A more targeted collateral recruitment endovascular therapy would also allow targeting of collateral cerebral network and therefore could have promising results.

AI in MT

The use of computing power further developed imaging that can be applied for stroke patient selection workflow, as well as identification of recanalization targets. However, using AI-based methods to improve the technical aspects of MT still requires further research but may represent the next step introduced into AIS therapy.

Presently, there is no quantitative method based on the clot composition and the treatment target that can aid in predicting the difficulty of endovascular treatment. Recently, it has been indicated that vessel architecture at the occlusion site in the form of the angle of interaction between the aspiration catheter and the clot is associated with successful recanalization [102, 103].

Another recent study also reported that the texture of the clot, or radiomic features (RFs), is predictive of recanalization following treatment with intravenous alteplase for AIS. This suggests that the extraction of pretherapeutic RF from radiological imaging may contain valuable information related to the composition of the clot, with an impact on the future success of MTB.

Attempts in another recent study to use pretherapeutic computed tomography (CT) to extract RF from the clot to investigate their capacity to predict the success of the MTB strategy were done in order to identify patients with first-attempt recanalization with thromboaspiration and to predict the overall number of passages with an MTB device required for successful recanalization [103].

By calculating the texture, size, shape, and higher order parameters of these clots and then developing a predictive model on a first training cohort, the authors highlighted the ability to identify patients with first-attempt recanalization following thromboaspiration in a second validation cohort.

Furthermore, in another study, Qiu et al. evaluated the value of radiomics in predicting the efficacy of intravenous alteplase in the treatment of patients with AIS. It was determined that radiomics analysis of heterogeneous thrombi texture was able to predict alteplase efficacy [104].

Over the past few years, evidence has also supported the idea that factors like the biological clot composition should be considered when choosing the fastest method to remove a clot. Recently, the use of AI to characterize the thrombus and guiding thrombectomy was utilized in Clotild®, a neurovascular guidewire equipped with the Sensome proprietary impedance sensor.

The latter allows the measurement of the electrophysiological characteristics of the surrounding tissues. Clotild® could categorize the thrombus occluding the cerebral blood vessel and support the neurointerventionist during mechanical thrombectomy for the treatment of ischemic stroke.

The CLOT OUT trial aims to demonstrate that using Clotild in humans is safe and can detect clot composition. The goal of this ongoing study is to evaluate the safety and the performance of the device. The electrophysiological measurements will be used to update Clotild®'s database and thus improve the prediction accuracy of the model in providing physicians with insights for mechanical thrombectomy.

References

1. Donkor ES. Stroke in the 21st century: a snapshot of the burden, epidemiology, and quality of life. Stroke Res Treat. 2018;2018:3238165.
2. Singer J, Gustafson D, Cummings C, Egelko A, Mlabasati J, Conigliaro A, et al. Independent ischemic stroke risk factors in older Americans: a systematic review. Aging. 2019;11:3392.
3. Catanese L, Tarsia J, Fisher M. Acute ischemic stroke therapy overview. Circ Res. 2017;120:541.
4. Shafie M, Yu W. Recanalization therapy for acute ischemic stroke with large vessel occlusion: where we are and what comes next? Transl Stroke Res. 2021;12:369.
5. Wallace AN, Kansagra AP, McEachern J, Moran CJ, Cross DT, Derdeyn CP. Evolution of endovascular stroke therapies and devices. Expert Rev Med Devices. 2016;13:263.
6. Rennert RC, Wali AR, Steinberg JA, Santiago-Dieppa DR, Olson SE, Pannell JS, et al. Epidemiology, natural history, and clinical presentation of large vessel ischemic stroke. Clin Neurosurg. 2019;85:S4.
7. Waqas M, Rai AT, Vakharia K, Chin F, Siddiqui AH. Effect of definition and methods on estimates of prevalence of large vessel occlusion in acute ischemic stroke: a systematic review and meta-analysis. J NeuroInterv Surg. 2020;12:260.
8. Lakomkin N, Dhamoon M, Carroll K, Singh IP, Tuhrim S, Lee J, et al. Prevalence of large vessel occlusion in patients presenting with acute ischemic stroke: a 10-year systematic review of the literature. J NeuroInterv Surg. 2019;11:241.
9. Smith WS, Lev MH, English JD, Camargo EC, Chou M, Johnston SC, et al. Significance of large vessel intracranial occlusion causing acute ischemic stroke and TIA. Stroke. 2009;40(12):3834.
10. Malhotra K, Gornbein J, Saver JL. Ischemic strokes due to large-vessel occlusions contribute disproportionately to stroke-related dependence and death: a review. Front Neurol. 2017;8:651.
11. Coutts SB, Eliasziw M, Hill MD, Scott JN, Subramaniam S, Buchan AM, et al. An improved scoring system for identifying patients at high early risk of stroke and functional impairment after an acute transient ischemic attack or minor stroke. Int J Stroke. 2008;3(1):3.
12. Hacke W, Kaste M, Fieschi C, Toni D, Lesaffre E, Von Kummer R, et al. Intravenous thrombolysis with recombinant tissue plasminogen activa-

tor for acute hemispheric stroke: the European Cooperative Acute Stroke Study (ECASS). JAMA J Am Med Assoc. 1995;274(13):1017.

13. Association of outcome with early stroke treatment: pooled analysis of ATLANTIS, ECASS, and NINDS rt-PA stroke trials. Lancet. 2004;363(9411):824.

14. Levine SR, Khatri P, Broderick JP, Grotta JC, Kasner SE, Kim D, et al. Review, historical context, and clarifications of the NINDS rt-PA stroke trials exclusion criteria: part 1: rapidly improving stroke symptoms. Stroke. 2013;44:2500.

15. Marler JR, Tilley BC, Lu M, Brott TG, Lyden PC, Grotta JC, et al. Early stroke treatment associated with better outcome: the NINDS rt-PA Stroke Study. Neurology. 2000;55(11):1649.

16. Emberson J, Lees KR, Lyden P, Blackwell L, Albers G, Bluhmki E, et al. Effect of treatment delay, age, and stroke severity on the effects of intravenous thrombolysis with alteplase for acute ischaemic stroke: a meta-analysis of individual patient data from randomised trials. Lancet. 2014;384(9958):1929.

17. Hacke W, Kaste M, Bluhmki E, Brozman M, Dávalos A, Guidetti D, et al. Thrombolysis with alteplase 3 to 4.5 hours after acute ischemic stroke. N Engl J Med. 2008;359(13):1317.

18. Lees KR, Bluhmki E, von Kummer R, Brott TG, Toni D, Grotta JC, et al. Time to treatment with intravenous alteplase and outcome in stroke: an updated pooled analysis of ECASS, ATLANTIS, NINDS, and EPITHET trials. Lancet. 2010;375(9727):1695.

19. Sandercock P, Wardlaw JM, Lindley RI, Dennis M, Cohen G, Murray G, et al. The benefits and harms of intravenous thrombolysis with recombinant tissue plasminogen activator within 6 h of acute ischaemic stroke (the third international stroke trial [IST-3]): a randomised controlled trial. Lancet. 2012;379(9834):2352.

20. Should thrombolytic therapy be the first-line treatment for acute ischemic stroke? N Engl J Med. 1997;337(18):1322.

21. Saqqur M, Uchino K, Demchuk AM, Molina CA, Garami Z, Calleja S, et al. Site of arterial occlusion identified by transcranial Doppler predicts the response to intravenous thrombolysis for stroke. Stroke. 2007;38(3):948.

22. del Zoppo GJ, Poeck K, Pessin MS, Wolpert SM, Furlan AJ, Ferbert A, et al. Recombinant tissue plasminogen activator in acute thrombotic and embolic stroke. Ann Neurol. 1992;32(1):78.

23. Bhatia R, Hill MD, Shobha N, Menon B, Bal S, Kochar P, et al. Low rates of acute recanalization with intravenous recombinant tissue plasminogen activator in ischemic stroke: real-world experience and a call for action. Stroke. 2010;41(10):2254.

24. Furlan AJ, Abou-Chebl A. The role of recombinant pro-urokinase (r-pro-UK) and intra-arterial thrombolysis in acute ischaemic stroke: the PROACT trials. Curr Med Res Opin. 2002;18(Suppl 2):s44–7.

25. Furlan A, Higashida R, Wechsler L, Gent M, Rowley H, Kase C, et al. Intra-arterial prourokinase for acute ischemic stroke. The PROACT II study: a randomized controlled trial. JAMA J Am Med Assoc. 1999;282(21):2003.

26. Smith WS, Sung G, Saver J, Budzik R, Duckwiler G, Liebeskind DS, et al. Mechanical thrombectomy for acute ischemic stroke: final results of the multi MERCI trial. Stroke. 2008;39(4):1205.

27. Smith WS, Sung G, Starkman S, Saver JL, Kidwell CS, Gobin YP, et al. Safety and efficacy of mechanical embolectomy in acute ischemic stroke: results of the MERCI trial. Stroke. 2005;36(7):1432.

28. Khatri P, Neff J, Broderick JP, Khoury JC, Carrozzella J, Tomsick T. Revascularization end points in stroke interventional trials: recanalization versus reperfusion in IMS-I. Stroke. 2005;36(11):2400.

29. Investigators PPST. The penumbra pivotal stroke trial: safety and effectiveness of a new generation of mechanical devices for clot removal in intracranial large vessel occlusive disease. Stroke. 2009;40(8):2761.

30. Ospel JM, Volny O, Jayaraman M, McTaggart R, Goyal M. Optimizing fast first pass complete reperfusion in acute ischemic stroke–the BADDASS approach (BAlloon guiDe with large bore distal access catheter with dual aspiration with Stent-retriever as Standard approach). Expert Rev Med Devices. 2019;16:955.

31. Saver JL, Jahan R, Levy EI, Jovin TG, Baxter B, Nogueira R, et al. SOLITAIRE™ with the intention for thrombectomy (SWIFT) trial: design of a randomized, controlled, multicenter study comparing the SOLITAIRE™ Flow Restoration device and the MERCI Retriever in acute ischaemic stroke. Int J Stroke. 2014;9(5):658.

32. Nogueira RG, Lutsep HL, Gupta R, Jovin TG, Albers GW, Walker GA, et al. Trevo versus Merci retrievers for thrombectomy revascularisation of large vessel occlusions in acute ischaemic stroke (TREVO 2): a randomised trial. Lancet. 2012;380(9849):1231.

33. Larrue V, Von Kummer R, Müller A, Bluhmki E. Risk factors for severe hemorrhagic transformation in ischemic stroke patients treated with recombinant tissue plasminogen activator: a secondary analysis of the European-Australasian Acute Stroke Study (ECASS II). Stroke. 2001;32(2):438.

34. Moreno A, Hernández-Fernández F. IMSIII, SYNTHESIS, and MR-RESCUE studies: the end of endovascular treatment for stroke? Radiologia. 2014;56(1):2.

35. Von Kummer R, Gerber J. IMS-3, SYNTHESIS, and MR RESCUE: no disaster, but down to earth. Clin Neuroradiol. 2013;23:1.

36. Berkhemer OA, Fransen PSS, Beumer D, van den Berg LA, Lingsma HF, Yoo AJ, et al. A randomized trial of intraarterial treatment for acute ischemic stroke. N Engl J Med. 2015;372(1):11.

37. Goyal M, Demchuk AM, Menon BK, Eesa M, Rempel JL, Thornton J, et al. Randomized assessment of rapid endovascular treatment of ischemic stroke. N Engl J Med. 2015;372(11):1019.

38. Symon L, Pasztor E, Branston NM. The distribution and density of reduced cerebral blood flow following acute middle cerebral artery occlusion: an experimental study by the technique of hydrogen clearance in baboons. Stroke. 1974;5(3):355.

39. Astrup J, Symon L, Branston NM, Lassen NA. Cortical evoked potential and extracellular k+ and h+ at critical levels of brain ischemia. Stroke. 1977;8(1):51.

40. Jones TH, Morawetz RB, Crowell RM, Marcoux FW, FitzGibbon SJ, DeGirolami U, et al. Thresholds of focal cerebral ischemia in awake monkeys. J Neurosurg. 1981;54(6):773.

41. Heiss WD, Graf R, Wienhard K, Löttgen J, Saito R, Fujita T, et al. Dynamic penumbra demonstrated by sequential multitracer PET after middle cerebral artery occlusion in cats. J Cereb Blood Flow Metab. 1994;14(6):892.

42. Baron JC, Bousser MG, Comar D, Soussaline F, Castaigne P. Noninvasive tomographic study of cerebral blood flow and oxygen metabolism in vivo potentials, limitations, and clinical applications in cerebral ischemic disorders. Eur Neurol. 1981;20(3):273.

43. Mintorovitch J, Moseley ME, Chileuitt L, Shimizu H, Cohen Y, Weinstein PR. Comparison of diffusion- and T2-weighted MRI for the early detection of cerebral ischemia and reperfusion in rats. Magn Reson Med. 1991;18(1):39.

44. Warach S, Dashe JF, Edelman RR. Clinical outcome in ischemic stroke predicted by early diffusion-weighted and perfusion magnetic resonance imaging: a preliminary analysis. J Cereb Blood Flow Metab. 1996;16(1):53.

45. Bykowski JL, Latour LL, Warach S. More accurate identification of reversible ischemic injury in human stroke by cerebrospinal fluid suppressed diffusion-weighted imaging. Stroke. 2004;35(5):1100.

46. Wittsack HJ, Ritzl A, Fink GR, Wenserski F, Siebler M, Seitz RJ, et al. MR imaging in acute stroke: diffusion-weighted and perfusion imaging parameters for predicting infarct size. Radiology. 2002;222(2):397.

47. Darby DG, Barber PA, Gerraty RP, Desmond PM, Yang Q, Parsons M, et al. Pathophysiological topography of acute ischemia by combined diffusion-weighted and perfusion MRI. Stroke. 1999;30(10):2043.

48. Scalzo F, Nour M, Liebeskind DS. Data science of stroke imaging and enlightenment of the penumbra. Front Neurol. 2015;6:8.

49. Zaro-Weber O, Moeller-Hartmann W, Heiss WD, Sobesky J. Maps of time to maximum and time to peak for mismatch definition in clinical stroke studies validated with positron emission tomography. Stroke. 2010;41(12):2817.

50. Takasawa M, Jones PS, Guadagno JV, Christensen S, Fryer TD, Harding S, et al. How reliable is perfusion MR in acute stroke? Validation and determination of the penumbra threshold against quantitative PET. Stroke. 2008;39(3):870.

51. Tan JC, Dillon WP, Liu S, Adler F, Smith WS, Wintermark M. Systematic comparison of perfusion-CT and CT-angiography in acute stroke patients. Ann Neurol. 2007;61(6):533.

52. Campbell BCV, Christensen S, Levi CR, Desmond PM, Donnan GA, Davis SM, et al. Comparison of computed tomography perfusion and magnetic resonance imaging perfusion-diffusion mismatch in ischemic stroke. Stroke. 2012;43(10):2648.

53. Lin L, Bivard A, Kleinig T, Spratt NJ, Levi CR, Yang Q, et al. Correction for delay and dispersion results in more accurate cerebral blood flow ischemic core measurement in acute stroke. Stroke. 2018;49(4):924.

54. Olivot JM, Mlynash M, Thijs VN, Kemp S, Lansberg MG, Wechsler L, et al. Relationships between infarct growth, clinical outcome, and early recanalization in diffusion and perfusion imaging for understanding stroke evolution (DEFUSE). Stroke. 2008;39(8):2257.

55. De Silva DA, Brekenfeld C, Ebinger M, Christensen S, Barber PA, Butcher KS, et al. The benefits of intravenous thrombolysis relate to the site of baseline arterial occlusion in the echoplanar imaging thrombolytic evaluation trial (EPITHET). Stroke. 2010;41(2):295.

56. Campbell BCV, Mitchell PJ, Kleinig TJ, Dewey HM, Churilov L, Yassi N, et al. Endovascular therapy for ischemic stroke with perfusion-imaging selection. N Engl J Med. 2015;372(11):1009.

57. Boyle K, Joundi RA, Aviv RI. An historical and contemporary review of endovascular therapy for acute ischemic stroke. Neurovasc Imaging. 2017;3(1):1.

58. Montoya S, Walters E, Mai N, Bhalla T. Endovascular embolectomy for emergent large vessel occlusion: a historical perspective. Am J Interv Radiol. 2017;1:2.

59. Ansari J, Triay R, Kandregula S, Adeeb N, Cuellar H, Sharma P. Endovascular intervention in acute ischemic stroke: history and evolution. Biomedicine. 2022;10(2)

60. Xiong Y, Huang CC, Fisher M, Hackney DB, Bhadelia RA, Selim MH. Comparison of automated CT perfusion softwares in evaluation of acute ischemic stroke. J Stroke Cerebrovasc Dis. 2019;28(12):104392.

61. Albers GW, Marks MP, Kemp S, Christensen S, Tsai JP, Ortega-Gutierrez S, et al. Thrombectomy for stroke at 6 to 16 hours with selection by perfusion imaging. N Engl J Med. 2018;378(8):708–18.

62. Rizvi A, Seyedsaadat SM, Murad MH, Brinjikji W, Fitzgerald ST, Kadirvel R, et al. Redefining 'success': a systematic review and meta-analysis comparing outcomes between incomplete and complete revascularization. J Neurointerv Surg. 2019;11(1):9–13.

63. Zaidat OO, Bozorgchami H, Ribó M, Saver JL, Mattle HP, Chapot R, et al. Primary results of the Multicenter ARISE II Study (analysis of revascularization in ischemic stroke with EmboTrap). Stroke. 2018;49(5):1107–15.
64. Yeo LLL, Jing M, Bhogal P, Tu T, Gopinathan A, Yang C, et al. Evidence-based updates to thrombectomy: targets, new techniques, and devices. Front Neurol. 2021;12:712527.
65. Kumar GGS, Nagesh C. Acute ischemic stroke: a review of imaging, patient selection, and management in the endovascular era. Part II: patient selection, endovascular thrombectomy, and postprocedure management. J Clin Interv Radiol ISVIR. 2018;02(03):169–83.
66. Sarraj A, Hassan AE, Grotta J, Sitton C, Cutter G, Cai C, et al. Optimizing patient selection for endovascular treatment in acute ischemic stroke (SELECT): a prospective, multicenter cohort study of imaging selection. Ann Neurol. 2020;87(3):419–33.
67. Saver JL, Fonarow GC, Smith EE, Reeves MJ, Grau-Sepulveda M, Pan W, et al. Time to treatment with intravenous tissue plasminogen activator and outcome from acute ischemic stroke. JAMA. 2013;309(23):2480.
68. Suzuki K, Kimura K, Takeuchi M, Morimoto M, Kanazawa R, Kamiya Y, et al. The randomized study of endovascular therapy with versus without intravenous tissue plasminogen activator in acute stroke with ICA and M1 occlusion (SKIP study). Int J Stroke. 2019;14(7):752–5.
69. Yang P, Zhang Y, Zhang L, Zhang Y, Treurniet KM, Chen W, et al. Endovascular thrombectomy with or without intravenous alteplase in acute stroke. N Engl J Med. 2020;382(21):1981–93.
70. Treurniet KM, LeCouffe NE, Kappelhof M, Emmer BJ, van Es ACGM, Boiten J, et al. MR CLEAN-NO IV: intravenous treatment followed by endovascular treatment versus direct endovascular treatment for acute ischemic stroke caused by a proximal intracranial occlusion-study protocol for a randomized clinical trial. Trials. 2021;22(1):141.
71. Goyal N, Tsivgoulis G, Malhotra K, Ishfaq MF, Pandhi A, Frohler MT, et al. Medical management vs mechanical thrombectomy for mild strokes: an international multicenter study and systematic review and meta-analysis. JAMA Neurol. 2020;77(1):16–24.
72. Jovin TG, Nogueira RG, Lansberg MG, Demchuk AM, Martins SO, Mocco J, et al. Thrombectomy for anterior circulation stroke beyond 6 h from time last known well (AURORA): a systematic review and individual patient data meta-analysis. Lancet. 2022;399(10321):249–58.
73. Nogueira RG, Jadhav AP, Haussen DC, Bonafe A, Budzik RF, Bhuva P, et al. Thrombectomy 6 to 24 hours after stroke with a mismatch between deficit and infarct. N Engl J Med. 2018;378(1):11–21.
74. Kim BJ, Menon BK, Kim JY, Shin DW, Baik SH, Jung C, et al. Endovascular treatment after stroke due to large vessel occlusion for patients presenting very late from time last known well. JAMA Neurol. 2020;78:21.

75. Yang D, Shi Z, Lin M, Zhou Z, Zi W, Wang H, et al. Endovascular retrograde approach may be a better option for acute tandem occlusions stroke. Interv Neuroradiol. 2019;25(2):194–201.

76. Lees KR, Emberson J, Blackwell L, Bluhmki E, Davis SM, Donnan GA, et al. Effects of alteplase for acute stroke on the distribution of functional outcomes: a pooled analysis of 9 trials. Stroke. 2016;47(9):2373–9.

77. Berkhemer OA, Borst J, Kappelhof M, Yoo AJ, van den Berg LA, Fransen PSS, et al. Extracranial carotid disease and effect of intra-arterial treatment in patients with proximal anterior circulation stroke in MR CLEAN. Ann Intern Med. 2017;166(12):867–75.

78. Rubiera M, Ribo M, Delgado-Mederos R, Santamarina E, Delgado P, Montaner J, et al. Tandem internal carotid artery/middle cerebral artery occlusion: an independent predictor of poor outcome after systemic thrombolysis. Stroke. 2006;37(9):2301–5.

79. Lockau H, Liebig T, Henning T, Neuschmelting V, Stetefeld H, Kabbasch C, et al. Mechanical thrombectomy in tandem occlusion: procedural considerations and clinical results. Neuroradiology. 2015;57(6):589–98.

80. Bekelis K, Missios S, MacKenzie TA, Tjoumakaris S, Jabbour P. Anesthesia technique and outcomes of mechanical thrombectomy in patients with acute ischemic stroke. Stroke. 2017;48(2):361–6.

81. McDonald JS, Brinjikji W, Rabinstein AA, Cloft HJ, Lanzino G, Kallmes DF. Conscious sedation versus general anaesthesia during mechanical thrombectomy for stroke: a propensity score analysis. J Neurointerv Surg. 2015;7(11):789–94.

82. Duloquin G, Graber M, Garnier L, Crespy V, Comby PO, Baptiste L, et al. Incidence of acute ischemic stroke with visible arterial occlusion. Stroke. 2020;51(7):2122–30.

83. Ospel JM, Menon BK, Demchuk AM, Almekhlafi MA, Kashani N, Mayank A, et al. Clinical course of acute ischemic stroke due to medium vessel occlusion with and without intravenous alteplase treatment. Stroke. 2020;51(11):3232–40.

84. Saber H, Narayanan S, Palla M, Saver JL, Nogueira RG, Yoo AJ, et al. Mechanical thrombectomy for acute ischemic stroke with occlusion of the M2 segment of the middle cerebral artery: a meta-analysis. J Neurointerv Surg. 2018;10(7):620–4.

85. Grøan M, Ospel J, Ajmi S, Sandset EC, Kurz MW, Skjelland M, et al. Time-based decision making for reperfusion in acute ischemic stroke. Front Neurol. 2021;12:728012.

86. Goyal M, McTaggart R, Ospel JM, van der Lugt A, Tymianski M, Wiest R, et al. How can imaging in acute ischemic stroke help us to understand tissue fate in the era of endovascular treatment and cerebroprotection? Neuroradiology. 2022;64(9):1697–707.

87. Kashani N, Cimflova P, Ospel JM, Singh N, Almekhlafi MA, Rempel J, et al. Endovascular device choice and tools for recanalization of medium vessel occlusions: insights from the MeVO FRONTIERS International Survey. Front Neurol. 2021;12:735899.

88. Teo YN, Sia CH, Tan BYQ, Mingxue J, Chan B, Sharma VK, et al. Combined balloon guide catheter, aspiration catheter, and stent retriever technique versus balloon guide catheter and stent retriever alone technique: a systematic review and meta-analysis. J Neurointerv Surg. 2022;15:127.

89. Pérez-García C, Moreu M, Rosati S, Simal P, Egido JA, Gomez-Escalonilla C, et al. Mechanical thrombectomy in medium vessel occlusions. Stroke. 2020;51(11):3224–31.

90. Pérez-García C, Rosati S, Gómez-Escalonilla C, López-Frías A, Arrazola J, Moreu M. MeVO SAVE technique: initial experience with the 167 cm long NeuroSlider 17 for a combined approach in medium vessel occlusions (MeVOs). J Neurointerv Surg. 2021;13(8):768–8.

91. McTaggart RA, Ospel JM, Psychogios MN, Puri AS, Maegerlein C, Lane KM, et al. Optimization of endovascular therapy in the neuroangiography suite to achieve fast and complete (expanded treatment in cerebral ischemia 2c-3) reperfusion. Stroke. 2020;51(7):1961–8.

92. Romano DG, Frauenfelder G, Napoletano R, Botto A, Locatelli G, Panza MP, et al. ADAPT with new catalyst 5 reperfusion catheter for distal M2 ischemic stroke: preliminary experience. World Neurosurg. 2020;135:e650–6.

93. Navia P, Larrea JA, Pardo E, Arce A, Martínez-Zabaleta M, Díez-González N, et al. Initial experience using the 3MAX cerebral reperfusion catheter in the endovascular treatment of acute ischemic stroke of distal arteries. J Neurointerv Surg. 2016;8(8):787–90.

94. Vargas J, Spiotta AM, Fargen K, Turner RD, Chaudry I, Turk A. Experience with A Direct Aspiration First Pass Technique (ADAPT) for thrombectomy in distal cerebral artery occlusions causing acute ischemic stroke. World Neurosurg. 2017;99:31–6.

95. Link TW, Santillan A, Patsalides A. Intra-arterial neuroprotective therapy as an adjunct to endovascular intervention in acute ischemic stroke: a review of the literature and future directions. Interv Neuroradiol. 2020;26(4):405–15.

96. Saver JL, Starkman S. Magnesium in the central nervous system. Adelaide (AU): University of Adelaide Press; 2011.

97. Fraser JF, Maniskas M, Trout A, Lukins D, Parker L, Stafford WL, et al. Intra-arterial verapamil post-thrombectomy is feasible, safe, and neuroprotective in stroke. J Cereb Blood Flow Metab. 2017;37(11):3531–43.

98. Konstas AA, Neimark MA, Laine AF, Pile-Spellman J. A theoretical model of selective cooling using intracarotid cold saline infusion in the human brain. J Appl Physiol (1985). 2007;102(4):1329–40.

99. Chen J, Liu L, Zhang H, Geng X, Jiao L, Li G, et al. Endovascular hypo-thermia in acute ischemic stroke: pilot study of selective intra-arterial cold saline infusion. Stroke. 2016;47(7):1933–5.

100. Choi JH, Marshall RS, Neimark MA, Konstas AA, Lin E, Chiang YT, et al. Selective brain cooling with endovascular intracarotid infusion of cold saline: a pilot feasibility study. AJNR Am J Neuroradiol. 2010;31(5):928–34.

101. Shuaib A, Bornstein NM, Diener HC, Dillon W, Fisher M, Hammer MD, et al. Partial aortic occlusion for cerebral perfusion augmentation. Stroke. 2011;42(6):1680–90.

102. Bernava G, Rosi A, Boto J, Brina O, Kulcsar Z, Czarnetzki C, et al. Direct thromboaspiration efficacy for mechanical thrombectomy is related to the angle of interaction between the aspiration catheter and the clot. J Neurointerv Surg. 2020;12(4):396–400.

103. Hofmeister J, Bernava G, Rosi A, Vargas MI, Carrera E, Montet X, et al. Clot-based radiomics predict a mechanical thrombectomy strategy for successful recanalization in acute ischemic stroke. Stroke. 2020;51(8):2488–94.

104. Qiu W, Kuang H, Nair J, Assis Z, Najm M, McDougall C, et al. Radiomics-based intracranial thrombus features on CT and CTA predict recanalization with intravenous alteplase in patients with acute ischemic stroke. AJNR Am J Neuroradiol. 2019;40(1):39–44.

Index

A

Activated clotting time (ACT), 122
Acute ischemic stroke (AIS), 87, 88,
    90, 91, 178–179
  AI in MT, 228
  contemporary strategies, 205,
    206, 212, 213
  image-guided stroke therapy,
    192, 193, 201, 203
  IV tPA, 217
  large ischemic core, 214, 215
  mechanical thrombectomy,
    184–187, 189, 191
  neuroprotection, 225–227
  paradigm shift, 5
  tandem occlusions, 218, 219
  thrombectomy, 219
Adjunctive aspiration devices, 40,
    43
Aneurysm, 6, 9
  screening, 164
Aneurysmal subarachnoid
    hemorrhage (aSAH), 149
Angiogenesis, 51
Ankle-brachial index (ABI), 160
Artificial intelligence (AI), 97, 163
Aspiration thrombectomy (AT), 206
Aspiration *vs.* Stent Retriever for
    Successful Revascularization
    (ASTER), 209

Augmented reality, 62, 63
Autosomal dominant polycystic
    kidney disease (ADPKD),
    155, 156

B

Balloon guide catheters (BGCs), 5,
    187, 211
Behcet's disease, 114
Blood-brain barrier (BBB), 35
Brain-computer interfaces (BCI),
    16, 18

C

Carotid artery disease (CAD), 71
Carotid artery stenting (CAS)
  distal embolic protection
    devices, 75, 76, 78, 79
  embolic protection devices, 72–75
  proximal embolic protection
    devices, 80
  technical innovations, 75
  trans carotid artery
    revascularization, 80–82
Carotid endarterectomy (CEA), 78
Carotid stenting, 74
Cerebral blood volume (CBV), 197
Cerebrospinal fluid diversion, 112

Cerebrospinal fluid-venous fistulas
    (CSFVFs), 12
Chronic subdural hematomas
    (cSDHs), 51, 52
Common carotid artery (CCA), 81
Computational fluid dynamics
    (CFD), 165
Computed tomography angiography
    (CTA), 203
Cone beam computed tomography
    (CBCT), 45
Connective tissue disorders, 159
CorPath GRX, 138
Cranioplasty, 64, 65
Craniopuncture, 36

D
Device precision, 135
Diffusion-weighted imaging (DWI),
    74, 195
Direct aspiration first-pass
    technique, 207
Disparity, 8
Distal access catheters (DAC), 211,
    222
Distal medium vessel occlusion
    (DMVO), 220
Door-to-needle times (DTN), 90
Dual antiplatelet therapy (DAPT),
    121, 124
Dutch intracerebral hemorrhage
    surgery trial (DIST), 44

E
Embolic protection devices (EPDs),
    72
Embolic System for Subacute and
    Chronic Subdural Hematoma
    (EMBOLISE), 57
Emergency departments (EDs), 89
Emergency medical services (EMS),
    88
Endoport-mediated evacuation, 38

Endoscope-assisted evacuation, 39
Endovascular-capable stroke care
    centers (ECCs), 8
Endovascular therapy (EVT), 93
Endovascular thrombectomy (EVT),
    95
Extracranial-intracranial (EC-IC)
    bypass, 61
    augmented reality, 63
    exoscope, 63
    peri-operative care, 61
    sonolucent cranioplasty, 64
    surgical techniques, 61

F
Familial intracranial aneurysm
    (FIA), 152
Fibromuscular dysplasia (FMD),
    161
Food and Drug Administration
    (FDA), 93
Forced aspiration thrombectomy
    (FAST), 207

H
Highly effective reperfusion
    evaluated in multiple
    endovascular stroke
    (HERMES), 200
Hydrocephalus, 15, 16

I
Idiopathic intracranial hypertension
    (IIH), 14, 104
    conservative, 110
    diagnosis, 108
    management, 110
    pathophysiology, 107
    prestenting evaluation, 116, 118,
        120
    surgical treatment, 112
    venous sinus stenting, 113, 114

Increased navigation, 135
Inflammation, 51
Inner diameter (ID), 207
Internal carotid artery (ICA), 53,
     178
International Study of Unruptured
     Intracranial Aneurysms
     (ISUIA 1), 149, 150
Intracranial aneurysms (IAs), 147,
     157
Intracranial atherosclerotic stenosis
     (ICAS), 212
Intracranial pressures (ICPs), 104,
     111

L

Large vessel occlusions (LVOs), 5,
     178, 179
Late-onset Pompe disease (LOPD),
     160
Leptomeningeal anastomosis
     (LMA), 228

M

Machine learning (ML), 148, 164
Mean-transit-time (MTT), 196, 197
Mechanical thrombectomy,
     183–185, 187
Medium-vessel occlusions
     (MeVOs), 220, 221
Middle cerebral artery (MCA), 178,
     181, 182, 184
Middle cerebral artery occlusion
     (MCAO), 193, 227
Middle meningeal artery (MMA),
     52–55, 57, 58, 63
Middle meningeal artery
     embolization (MMAE), 52
Middle-sized vessel occlusions
     (MVOs), 178
Minimally invasive surgery (MIS),
     27–28

Moyamoya, 62
Myocardial infarction (MI), 74

N

N-butyl cyanoacrylate (NBCA), 54
Neurointervention, 4, 5, 9
Neurologic emergency department,
     89
Neuroprotection, 224
Neurovascular robotics, 135

O

Optic nerve sheath fenestration
     (ONSF), 105, 111, 121

P

Picture archiving and communication
     system (PACS), 92
Poly-methyl-methylacrylate
     (PMMA), 64
Postoperative monitoring, 66
Primary motor cortex (PMC), 63
Pseudotumor cerebri (PTC), 104

R

Randomized controlled trials
     (RCTs), 72
Recombinant tissue plasminogen
     activator (rtPA), 37
Recombinant tissue-type
     plasminogen activator
     (r-tPA), 179, 180
Relative cerebral blood volume
     (rCBV), 196
Robotic-assisted endovascular
     intervention, 136, 138
  CorPath GRX, 139, 140
  limitations, 142, 143
  telerobotic intervention, 141,
     142

Robotics, 10
Rupture risk, 166

S
Single nucleotide polymorphisms
　(SNPs), 153
Spontaneous intracerebral
　hemorrhage (ICH)
　endoscope-assisted evacuation,
　　39, 40
　multiple animal models, 35
　trial, 28
Stereotactic evacuation, 37
Stroke, 177
　care, 7, 9
　champion, 92, 93
Subarachnoid hemorrhage (SAH),
　149, 152
Superior sagittal sinus (SSS), 119
Surgiscope, 45
Symptomatic intracranial
　hemorrhage (sICH), 92

T
Telerobotic Intervention, 141
Tenecteplase, 91, 95
Thrombolysis in cerebral infarction
　(TICI), 204

Thrombolysis in cerebral ischemia
　(TICI), 188
Thrombolysis in myocardial
　infarction score (TIMI), 204
Time-to-peak (TTP), 197
Tobacco consumption, 158
Traditional emergency department
　(TED), 90
Transcarotid approach (TCAR), 71
Transcarotid artery revascularization
　(TCAR), 72, 73, 81
Transfemoral approach (TFA), 9
Transient ischemic attack (TIA), 161
Transradial approaches (TRA), 9
Transverse sinus stenosis, 105, 113

U
Unruptured intracranial aneurysms
　(UIAs), 148, 149

V
Venous sinus outflow obstruction
　(VSOO), 106
Venous sinus stenting, 105, 106
　complications, 124, 125
　prestenting evaluation, 116, 120,
　　121
　technique, 122–124

Printed in the United States
by Baker & Taylor Publisher Services